KT-158-355

Sociology for Social Workers and Probation Officers

Viviene E. Cree

U.W.E.L
LEARNING RESOURCES

ACC No. 2301711   CLASS 803

CONTROL
0415150159

DATE
9 MAR 2004   SITE WV

301.
0243
62
CRE

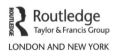

Routledge
Taylor & Francis Group

LONDON AND NEW YORK

First published 2000
by Routledge
11 New Fetter Lane, London EC4P 4EE

Simultaneously published in the USA and Canada
by Routledge
29 West 35th Street, New York, NY 10001

Routledge is an imprint of the Taylor & Francis Group

Reprinted 2002, 2004

© 2000 Viviene E. Cree

Typeset in Garamond by Taylor & Francis Books Ltd
Printed and bound in Great Britain by MPG Books Ltd, Bodmin

All rights reserved. No part of this book may be reprinted
or reproduced or utilised in any form or by any electronic,
mechanical, or other means, now known or hereafter
invented, including photocopying and recording, or in any
information storage or retrieval system, without permission in
writing from the publishers.

British Library Cataloguing in Publication Data
A catalogue record for this book is available from the British Library

Library of Congress Cataloging in Publication Data
Cree, Vivienne E., 1954–
    Sociology of social workers and probation officers / Viviene E. Cree
    P.   cm.
    1. Social Service – Sociological aspects. 2. Probation – Sociological
    aspects. 3. Sociology. I. Title.
HV41.C74 2000
301–dc2   99–31463
                               CIP

ISBN 0–415–15015–9 (hbk)
ISBN 0–415–15016–7 (pbk)

For Kate

Contents

Preface

Every year more and more sociological texts fill the bookshops and libraries: basic introductions, heavy theoretical tomes and a bewildering array of texts on the sociology of the family, crime, employment, education, feminist perspectives and even a sociology of social work. For the social work or probation student with little or no background knowledge of sociology, the field must seem vast and forbidding. With a limited budget to spend on books, which does the student choose to buy: the specialist or the generic text, the introduction or the book on theory? Just as important, how does the student make the connections between sociological knowledge and day-to-day practice in social work and probation?

Sociology for Social Workers and Probation Officers fills a gap in the sociological/social work literature by providing an introduction to sociological ideas and sociological research while at the same time considering the relevance and application of these ideas and concepts to practice with service-users. It examines a range of sociological concepts that are central to an understanding of the context in which practice takes place, and it argues that sociological insight can inform and improve practice today. Howe (1987: 166) makes a useful distinction between theories *for* social work and theories *of* social work. Theories *for* social work help to explain people and their situations and to inform practice; theories *of* social work say something about social work itself: what is it? what is it for? what should it be like? This book is a sociology *for* social workers and probation officers, looking at the ways in which sociological understandings might inform and improve practice.

Sociology for Social Workers and Probation Officers explores the sociological ideas that influence practice with service-users across *all* service-user groups: children and families, adult and community care, criminal justice and probation. The profession of social work in the UK has become increasingly fragmented and specialised in recent years. The probation service has withdrawn from social work training in England and Wales. What were previously social work tasks in community care are now increasingly being carried out by other professional groups, including nurses and health visitors. It is becoming more difficult to identify 'social work' as something distinct from the workings of care management, advocacy, child protection and criminal justice. This does not, however, detract from the main purpose of this book. *Sociology for Social Workers and Probation Officers* remains relevant to those working in social work, social services and probation, whatever their job title and organisational setting. I have chosen to continue to use the generic term 'social work' throughout the book for the sake of clarity, fully aware that this concept is likely to continue to shift in the years ahead.

Aims of the book

Sociology for Social Workers and Probation Officers will examine key sociological themes within social work and probation practice, drawing attention to the often unexplored assumptions and ideas on which practice is based. The focus of each chapter will be on developing understanding of the context within which practice operates (individual, family, and community), while at the same time analysing fundamental ideas in social work and probation (about childhood and adolescence, crime and deviance, care and control). I will present different theoretical positions and encourage readers to reach their own views of the usefulness and implications of holding certain positions. I will also endeavour to take an anti-discriminatory stance, pointing out the racism, sexism, heterosexism and disablism that permeate classical and present-day sociological and social work knowledge and practice.

The book is more than simply a review of sociological literature, or a restatement of sociological theories. On the contrary, it is my intention to build and develop new knowledge about social work practice – knowledge which reflects sociological issues and concerns. I believe that this is not only the most helpful way to work with service-users, but that it also may help to guard against cynicism, pessimism and 'burn-out' in our work, by encouraging us to look beyond immediate personal distress and the confusion of people's lives. Mills (1959) describes this as a 'sociological imagination'. He writes:

The first fruit of this imagination ... is the idea that the individual can understand his own experience and gauge his own fate only by locating himself within his period, that he can know his own chances in life only by becoming aware of those of all individuals in his circumstances. In many ways it is a terrible lesson; in many ways a magnificent one.

(1959: 5)

Mills' language may seem rather dated, but the issues he is raising are as relevant today as when they were written. Mills urges that we develop a self-consciousness about ourselves and our lives; that we go about with our eyes wide open, willing to ask questions and to make relevant connections between our experiences and those of others, between 'personal troubles of milieu' and 'public issues of social structure' (1959: 8). The study of sociology, then, is not simply an intellectual exercise. It is a way of thinking and being that encourages us to ask questions and strive to make changes in the society in which we live.

Structure of the book

The book begins with a chapter that sets out the key sociological perspectives which will be developed throughout the book. Thereafter, each chapter follows a similar structure. Chapter 2 explores the family, giving attention to the ways in which ideas about the family (what it is and what people think it should be) influence professional practice with families today. Chapters 3 and 4 discuss childhood and youth, both central to social work practice with children and young people, whether they are perceived as 'troubled' or 'troublesome'. Chapters 5 and 6 consider sociologically the dual aspects of community care: community and caring. Chapter 7 is the longest chapter in the book; it explores ideas of crime, deviance and social control. Each chapter is fully referenced so that readers may either draw on the material as set, or go to primary sources for further elaboration of specific themes or ideas. Each chapter also finishes with a small number of recommended texts that will give readers a good introduction to the subject under consideration.

Bernardes (1997: xvii) argues that a textbook is where things start, not where they finish. *Sociology for Social Workers and Probation Officers* should be regarded as a springboard for social work and probation students, practice teachers and practitioners. It aims to identify and consider sociological concepts that have a direct bearing on practice across all its current specialist areas, including children and families' social work, criminal justice and probation, and adult and community care. It cannot, however, cover the whole field of sociology. In the interests of writing a readable and manageable text, I have had to make decisions about what to include, and what to leave out. This has proved extraordinarily difficult, and even up to the last moments of pulling the manuscript together, I have continued to read and draw in new material. What finally appears in the book is a selection of some of the material that I have found interesting and relevant to my overall objective. I hope that readers will find the selection useful, but that they will also feel able to take forward the ideas and issues raised by reading more widely and by making connections with their own experience.

Dr Viviene E. Cree
Edinburgh
April 1999

Acknowledgements

This book would not have been possible without the support and encouragement, ideas and suggestions of a number of people. First, thanks go to my partner Colin MacDonald and my friend and colleague from the University of Glasgow, Dr Kate Cavanagh. Both have read the book and made helpful comments on early versions of the text. Second, I would like to thank my colleagues at the University of Edinburgh, particularly Professor Lorraine Waterhouse and Bill Whyte, who both gave input and feedback as requested. Third, my thanks go to Heather Gibson at Routledge, who has remained enthusiastic about the book throughout the life of the project. Finally, I wish to acknowledge the contributions and insights of generations of social work students who have raised my awareness and sharpened my thinking by their questions and their discussion at sociology lectures over my time at the University of Edinburgh.

1 Sociological perspectives

Definitions

What is sociology?

The discipline of sociology, according to Macionis and Plummer (1997: 4), is 'the systematic, sceptical study of human society'. It is a subject that is both ordinary and extraordinary. It starts with something we implicitly know about, that is, the relationship between ourselves as individuals and society. It then sets out to examine this afresh, to encourage us to think about and 'unpack' our common-sense assumptions and attitudes about society and our place in it. It does so by, at times, taking a broad view, looking at structures and institutions within society now and across history. At other times, it takes a microscopic view, interrogating the minute processes and relationships that make up our daily lives. From this we can see that we are the first subjects in the sociological enterprise, but we are also members of a particular society, born at a given historical moment with a specific gender, class, ethnic, cultural and racial grouping. It is only by stepping outside our own lives and experiences that we can begin to see the patterns and the systems that govern our existence. C. Wright Mills (1959) calls this process of stepping-outside, 'the sociological imagination'. He writes:

> The task of sociology is that people should be enabled to grasp the relations between themselves and the way in which their society operates ... The sociological imagination enables us to grasp history and biography and the relations between the two in society.
>
> (Mills 1959: 8)

What is society?

If sociology is about analysing society, then this begs the question what is 'society'? Classical sociology assumed that there was something which we could point to and recognise as 'society' or even as 'Society'. In the European and North American context, it was the development of urban, industrial, capitalist society which was at the heart of the sociological enterprise: the sociologist's job was to explain the changes that were taking place and analyse the ways in which people were located in the new, 'modern'[1] society. Marx, Weber and Durkheim were all engaged in this enterprise in different ways. 'Modern' for early sociologists signified progress, scientific reasoning and enlightened thinking; it also encapsulated the idea of a loss of traditional values and ways of life. 'Modern' was everything that 'primitive' was not:

'Primitive' society   'Modern' society

Feudal	Capitalist
Agrarian	Industrial
Rural	Urban
Simple	Complex
Religious	Secular
Faith	Science
Superstition	Reasoning
Tradition	Progress

In more recent years, the idea of society as a unitary phenomenon has been severely criticised. Pluralist approaches present society as a mosaic of competing worlds; power is seen as spread across a wide range of social locations, and the task of sociology is to investigate the different interest groups and coalitions that come together at different points in time (Marsh *et al.* 1996: 192). 'Postmodern' perspectives take this further, emphasising the contingent nature of our existence and the chaotic, unexpected characteristics of late capitalist society (see, for example, the work of Foucault). Society is now perceived as complex and fragmented: just as we have more than one identity, so there are many competing societies within which we live and move. 'Modern' society is again understood in opposition, this time to 'postmodern' society:

'Modern' society   'Postmodern' society

Capitalist	Post-capitalist
Industrial	Post-industrial

Urban	Global
Complex	Fragmented
Secular	Pluralist
Knowledge	Relativity
Scientific facts	Beliefs
Truths	Contingencies

Sociology's customary concern with issues of structure and power has not, however, disappeared. On the contrary, sociologists today maintain that the identities and societies which we inhabit continue to be structured by wider experiences of class, gender, 'race', ethnicity, age, sexuality and disability, and by the power relations that flow from these (see, for example, the writings of Bauman, 1990 and 1992).

Social work and sociology

The relationship between social work and sociology has been a changing one, reflecting broader debates about the nature of knowledge and the understanding of theory and practice within both subjects.

Today departments of social work and sociology in universities and colleges are likely to be separate units with distinct approaches and different personnel. This was not always the case. When the Charity Organisation Society in Britain began the first academic institution devoted to the training of social workers in 1903, they named it the School of Sociology (Smith 1965). This tells us a great deal about the ways in which sociology and social work were conceptualised in the early years of the twentieth century. Sociology and social work were seen as two sides of one coin: social reform in Britain and the United States was based on the assumption that sociology and social work went hand-in-hand, as the work of Charles Booth, Beatrice Webb and Seebohm Rowntree illustrates. They believed that, in charting the living conditions of the urban poor, their wider project for social reform and social welfare might be realised. This was the promise of the 'modern' age: that through scientific discovery and rational investigation, the 'truth' might be uncovered, which would lead to an improvement in the workings of society and in the lives of individuals.

Social work was not, however, only concerned in its early years with large-scale social change. It was also routinely concerned with finding individual solutions to individual problems. The work of the Charity Organisation Society focused on individuals and their families, but situated in the context of their social networks. Mary Richmond, writing what became a textbook for social work practice in Britain and the United States, suggested that sociology offered practical guidance for carrying out the social work task by helping social workers to make assessments of the situations which they faced. Richmond stressed the importance of *social* factors in the social worker's understanding of the individual, and she urged the collecting of 'social facts' or 'evidence' as a foundation of assessment (Richmond 1917). (This is highly reminiscent of Durkheim's *The Rules of Sociological Method*, first published in 1895, in which he argues that the study of society is made possible by the collection of 'social facts'.)

The relationship between social work and sociology has remained a live and contested issue for social work. Writing in 1931, Robert MacIvor argued in *The Contribution of Sociology to Social Work* that, although sociology has no direct therapeutic implications for social work, it nevertheless provides 'the basis for the development of that social philosophy which must integrate the thinking of the social worker, which must control the direction and illuminate the goal of his activity' (quoted in Leonard 1966: 15). In practice, sociology has not provided social work with the underpinning social philosophy envisaged by MacIvor. Instead, the knowledge-base of social work over the last 60 years or so has been dominated largely by ideas and practices that have their origins in psychological perspectives (Cree 1995, Yelloly 1980). Sociological voices have remained on the edge of mainstream social work theory and knowledge, struggling to be heard above the predominantly individual, psychological and correctional discourses in social work. Sociological ideas did, however, play an important part in social work thinking in the 1970s, when the radical social work movement looked to sociology to explain the workings of state capitalism and the role of social work within the welfare state (see Bailey and Brake 1975). The development of a feminist critique and black perspectives in social work in the 1980s also drew on a sociological framework of understanding (see Dominelli and McLeod 1989, Hanmer and Statham 1988). But these ideas came under open attack in the 1980s and 1990s as part of a concerted attempt to discredit what were seen as 'left wing' influences on social work practice. Educational institutions and social work agencies were pilloried for their 'political correctness'; at the same time there were strong indications that the teaching of sociology might be removed altogether from social work education (Jones 1997). Social work educators and practitioners have resisted such developments, and sociological ideas remain part of the knowledge-base of social work, albeit alongside psychological perspectives (CCETSW 1995).

My own assessment of the relationship between sociology and social work is a positive and realistic one. Sociology cannot be assumed to offer a single set of solutions to either society's or social work's problems, not least because there are myriad sociological perspectives and a host of possible ways of conceptualising the individual and society. The 'modern' dream of enlightened progress and increasing rationality has been exposed as a myth: theory, knowledge and ideas are all contextually and historically specific, conditional and open to challenge. Over and above this, theory, knowledge and ideas can never be assumed to be neutral, value-free or apolitical. Foucault (1977) has demonstrated that knowledge, ideas and practice are sites in which power is acted out; as a consequence, what we hold to be 'true', in terms of our understanding of the society in which we live, both reflects the state of contestation which is inevitably at the heart of the sociological discourse and at the same time sets the parameters and structures of that sociological enterprise. Sociology, then, in common with social work and all the social and human sciences, may be regarded as an integral part of the process through which society investigates, controls and manages (or using Foucault's terminology, 'disciplines') its citizens. In this way, both sociology and social work construct the 'individual' (and in the same way, the family and the community) of whom the discipline then speaks (Gubrium and Silverman 1989).

This is why social work needs a sociological imagination. Social work's central purpose is to work on behalf of society to help those individuals and groups who are vulnerable and marginalised. But the problems which these individuals and groups face may not be of their own making: the origins and maintenance of what are presented to us daily as individual problems may lie in structures of inequality in society. Explanations are therefore likely to be found not in individual psychology or in biology but in social practices and social structures. Social workers must be able to understand the connections between individual problems and society: between 'personal troubles and the public issues of social structure' (Mills 1959: 8). If social workers cannot make these connections, there is a very real risk that, by pathologising and blaming individuals and families, they will perpetuate the oppression and discrimination which characterise the lives of users of social work services. In Jones' words, they will 'abandon their clients' [2] (1997: 33).

Sociological insights may be useful at an institutional and organisation level, as well as at the level of knowledge creation. Questions raised by sociological thinking may provide planners and managers of services with a framework for reviewing structures and systems which operate so that services can be planned and managed in a thoughtful and critical way. A sociological imagination may allow planners to look at a situation from the vantage points of competing systems of interpretation (Berger 1967). Better still, a historical sociological analysis may allow decision-makers to see the connections between personal activity and social organisation as it is continuously constructed in time (Abrams 1982).

This does not, however, suggest that social work is a kind of applied sociology, or that social workers can lead service-users to a new kind of consciousness through sociological understanding. As Davies wryly comments, 'sociologists ask questions; social workers must act as though they have answers.' The social worker, he continues 'is a revolutionary irrelevance – a mere employee in the welfare industry, with a range of quite specific skills to learn, tasks to perform, services to deliver, a professional identity to maintain, and a career to pursue' (1991: 7). But even within this circumscribed existence, the social worker has choices to make and a degree of autonomy of action. It is crucial that social workers act in a way that seeks to empower, not oppress, service-users (Braye and Preston-Shoot 1995: 8). At the same time, social workers must be encouraged to reflect on their own experiences and their own practice, not just in the narrow sense of developing skills, but in terms of understanding the role of social work within the state and the scope they may (or may not) have for negotiation and creativity within this. Social workers must learn to 'unpack' or deconstruct their attitudes and values and to examine the theoretical frameworks that structure their thinking and practice. They must begin to see the connections and interplay between themselves and others, as well as between others and their own social structures. This is expressed well by Sullivan, who states that 'sociological theory and sociological imagination form invaluable weapons in the struggle for critical and reflective social work practice' (1987: 155).[3]

To argue that social workers need a sociological understanding does not, of course, imply that other understandings are unimportant. Social workers should also understand the influence of psychological approaches on social work: psycho-dynamic, developmental, cognitive and behavioural. There are occasions where sociological and psychological explanations will be at variance with one another, for example in some studies of crime and deviant behaviour (see Practice Example at end of this chapter). There are also areas of overlap between the interests and concerns of psychologists and those of sociologists, particularly around socialisation and the family. In recent years, postmodernist and post-structuralist sociologists have become increasingly interested in subject areas which in the past were considered the domain of psychology:

sexuality, identity, even psychoanalytic approaches (see Ramazanoglu 1993, Ussher 1997).

Social work is itself a subject of sociological interest, generating a large number of studies of professionalisation and bureaucratisation, organisation, managerialism, social work practice, social work education, and social control in social work (for example, Hearn and Parkin 1987, Hearn 1996, Heraud 1970, Day 1987, Davies 1991, Sibeon 1991, Dominelli 1997).

Summary

In conclusion, sociology offers social work the opportunity to explore meanings beneath taken-for-granted assumptions about behaviour, action and social structure. It offers a knowledge and value base which is not rooted in individual pathology but instead seeks to understand individuals in the context of the broader structures which make up their lives (including social class, gender, age, 'race' and ethnicity) and the historical moment within which they are living. Sociology also offers critical, reflective tools for social work practice. Sullivan (1987: 173–4) describes these as three-fold:

1   the ability to take on the role of the outsider – to take a greater distance from the traumatic situations social workers often face than is often possible when we take the role of friend or contemporary;
2   the skills of disengaging from our own existential concerns in order to better understand the phenomena we are observing;
3   the ability to place the phenomenon confronting us in the context of the social and economic as well as in the context of the individual and family.

The discipline of sociology

The emergence of Western sociology

The foundation of sociology as an academic discipline is usually attributed to Auguste Comte (1798–1857). He is credited with inventing the name 'sociology' and also the term 'positivism', although the study of society as a historical and empirical object had begun much earlier, in what has become known as the seventeenth- and eighteenth-century Enlightenment.[4] Building on the work of Scottish and French Enlightenment philosophers and economists, Comte argued that the search for order and progress in the social world would be achieved not by investigation of human nature, but by scientific experimentation and by analysis of what he called 'social facts'.[5] Of course sociological ideas (about social differentiation, social inequality, conflict, human nature and society) were not in themselves new, and had been around at least since the philosophical writings of classical Greece (Ritzer 1992). But it is to the end of the nineteenth century that we must look to find the broad expansion of sociology as a discipline in its own right. Sociology advanced at this time out of a need to understand the changes which had accompanied the process of 'modernisation' in society (see p.2). Urbanisation, industrialisation and the revolution in France had brought in their wake an increase in crime, deviance, suicide and disorder. There was a crisis in religious faith, as new ideas from science challenged established beliefs and practices. Liberalism was seen as failing to cope with the challenges of the 'modern' world. Sociologists set out to describe and explain the changes and to offer new ways of understanding the relations between the individual and society (Rose 1993). The three 'founders' of sociological theory, Emile Durkheim (1858–1917), Max Weber (1864–1920) and Karl Marx (1818–1883), were all engaged in this enterprise, but from different perspectives and reaching very different conclusions. Bilton *et al.* offer a useful outline of the main ideas and beliefs encompassed in the 'modernist project':

> Modernity involves a distinctive position regarding the nature of knowledge and the part it can and should play in the lives of human beings and human societies. Modernists are committed to the idea that it is possible to attain rational, verifiable, cumulative knowledge of society, to construct from that theories through which social phenomena can be represented and explained, and that competing theories or narratives can be evaluated by an appeal to logic and the testing of their claims – that is, a particular theory or narrative can be 'right' ... Moreover, modernism involves belief in the idea of *progress through knowledge* – that the accumulation of knowledge can be acted on to emancipate human beings, to enrich their lives, improve society and humanity generally, and achieve progress and better futures.
>
> (1996: 450)

Sociology has continued to develop (as we will see), sometimes building on early approaches and at other times seeking to find new ways of making sense of the set of problems and relations which are part and parcel of living in a so-called 'modern' or even 'postmodern' society. It is important to stress here that sociology is not one subject upon which all sociologists will agree. Instead, it is replete with disputes and disagreements. Sociologists are constantly in the process of redefining, contesting, changing and developing sociological knowledge. There can be no end-point in this, as sociologists rework old theories and ideas and introduce new ways of thinking which engage with and challenge existing knowledge.

Sociological frameworks

An overview

At their most simple, classical sociological theories can be divided into two broad frameworks. On the one hand, there are *structural* theories, which share a macro-level orientation and are concerned with large-scale questions about what holds society together and how it changes over time (see, for example, the writings of Durkheim and Marx). On the other hand, there are *interpretive* or *action* theories, which offer a micro-level orientation and focus on social interaction in specific situations (demonstrated in the work of Weber) (Macionis and Plummer 1997: 22). Within the structural framework, two competing approaches can be identified: structural-consensus theories, such as functionalism, and structural-conflict theories which draw on a Marxist, or 'conflict', paradigm. Functionalism is a framework that conceptualises society as 'a complex system whose parts work together to promote solidarity and stability' (Macionis and Plummer 1997: 19–20). Talcott Parsons' work illustrates this approach. The conflict paradigm, in contrast, imagines society 'as an arena of inequality that generates conflict and change' (ibid.). There are many sociologists who take a conflict approach as their starting-point, including Ralf Dahrendorf.

More recent sociological approaches that reflect *critical* ideas have attempted to blend structural and interpretive theories to bring about a better understanding of the relationship between the individual and society. Habermas, for example, has argued that neither approach gives a satisfactory base for social theory on its own; instead, both are different aspects of social reality (Fulcher and Scott 1999: 60). In addition, feminist and black sociologists have drawn attention to the absences from conventional sociology: the voices and perspectives of women and black people (as well as those of disabled people, older people, gay men and lesbian women) have been almost entirely

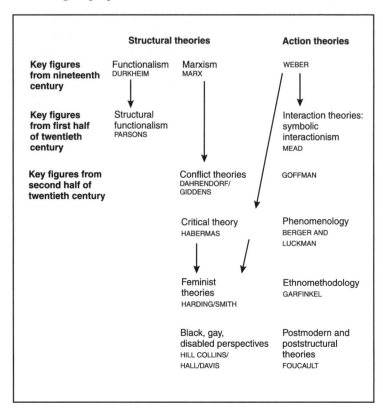

Figure 1.1 Sociological perspectives

missing from the frameworks and analyses of conventional Western sociology.

Figure 1.1 provides an illustration of the main developments of sociological perspectives and names some key contributors to sociological knowledge.

The functionalist paradigm

A functionalist approach, illustrated in the writing of Durkheim and the standard sociological approach between the 1920s and the 1950s, sets out to understand how society holds together and how it changes over time, particularly in the context of the shift from feudalism to industrial society. Functionalism offers an equilibrium model of society: society is conceived as a complete system made up of interconnected and interdependent parts, all working together to achieve the maintenance and continuity of the whole. Comparisons are frequently drawn with biology, as Bilton *et al.* explain:

> The health of an organism depends on all the organs that make up the system working properly together, each organ performing a necessary *function* for the organism's health.
>
> (1996: 82)

As all the parts of the body work together to maintain the body, so it is with institutions in society (that is, the family, education, religion, political systems, the economy), whose 'function' it is to contribute to the maintenance and survival of the wider social system. Social order and individual well-being are seen as one and the same thing: individuals need the control and regulation that keeps society in order, because without it they are unhappy and unfulfilled. Happiness and social order are therefore both based on a core of shared values.

Durkheim is widely regarded as the principal figure in the establishment of the functionalist tradition in sociology. Durkheim's primary objective was to create a new understanding of society, as a corrective to the biological and psychological approaches of his day, which saw human behaviour largely in terms of the actions of individuals. Durkheim argued that human behaviour should be understood in terms of social structures, not individual motives or choices. Social structures are 'social facts' that have an objective reality beyond individuals (Durkheim called this '*sui generis*'). Social facts are collective ways of thinking, feeling and acting that are acquired through learning and training and that constrain and regulate our thoughts, emotions and behaviour. Some social facts are institutions (beliefs and modes of behaviour); others are collective representations (shared ways of thinking, such as myths, legends and religious beliefs). Some are codified, written down in laws and religious texts; others are less overt but no less powerful. (See Fulcher and Scott 1999: 35.) Macionis and Plummer explain this simply:

> Durkheim recognised that society exists beyond ourselves. Society is more than the individuals who compose it; society has a life of its own that stretches beyond our personal experiences. It was here

long before we are born, it makes claims on us while we are alive, and it will remain long after we are gone.

(1997: 88)

Durkheim (1938) argued that sociologists should treat social facts as 'things' and study them as such; if sociology was to be a science, it had to collect evidence in exactly the same way as the physical sciences, through the direct observation and investigation of social facts. (This is the essence of what is called a 'positivist' approach.) Durkheim's (1952) study of suicide is regarded as the pioneering piece of positivist sociology (Bilton *et al.* 1996: 84). Here he demonstrated that suicide rates were significantly higher amongst those people who were less well-integrated socially. This shows that society affects even the most personal of our actions: that suicide is, in fact, a *social* act.

The structural functionalist sociologist who has had most impact on social policy and on social work theory and practice is Talcott Parsons (1902–1979). Parsons (1951) understood the structure of society as a normative framework, consisting of 'the norms that define the expectations and obligations that govern people's actions and so shape their social realities' (Fulcher and Scott 1999: 48). At the heart of this normative framework are agreed definitions of role and behaviour, with each person playing their part in a complex social division of labour. For example, the roles of husband, wife, and child in a family are seen as complementary and separate (1949). Parsons argues that people learn how to behave (that is, they learn what the normative expectations and obligations are) through socialisation. This is possible because cultural values and social norms are seen as widely shared by members of society (Fulcher and Scott 1999: 49).

There are, as we can see, a number of implicit assumptions in a functionalist approach, all of which have been challenged by subsequent conflict and pluralist perspectives. First, it is assumed that for society to function, all the parts (institutions) are working to the same end: that there is some kind of compatibility between institutions. This leads to a second assumption, that there is a level of agreement about means and goals in society, a value consensus, which is to a minimum degree held by all. Finally, there is an underlying assumption that order and stability are essential for the survival of society and that social control must play a part in maintaining that order. Durkheim, for example, believed that order and regulation in industrial society needed to be strengthened through effective socialisation, so that individuals would learn how to behave and to think appropriately. There is no notion here of the choices and behaviours of individuals in society; of the ways in which different groups in society may have their own values and perspectives which are at odds with those of 'mainstream' society; or the impact of differential power and opportunities for setting the core agenda in society.

The Marxist paradigm

Marxist perspectives, like functionalism, set out to explain how society works and how change has come about from feudal to industrial society. Marxist approaches also begin with the starting point that society is best understood as an objective whole and that individual actions should be explored in terms of the social structure in which they are located. Society is no longer seen as a consensus, however: contradictions are held to be endemic within capitalism, just as conflict between diverse and opposing interest groups in society is held to be inevitable. Social control is seen here as functional only in terms of propping up existing privileges and inequalities within society. Marxist approaches were increasingly influential in sociology during the 1970s.

Karl Marx, like Durkheim, was inspired to build a science of society. But he did not describe himself as a sociologist, and his ideas were not picked up until the next generation of sociologists (Fulcher and Scott 1999: 30). Marx sought to understand not simply the development of industrial society, but rather the development of capitalist society. He argued that industrialisation had transformed a small number of people into a class of private property owners (capitalists) and most of the rest of the population into industrial workers (the 'proletariat'). He saw an inevitable conflict in this, as capitalists sought to maximise profits and keep down costs, and workers sought to increase their wages and their standards of living. (Macionis and Plummer 1997: 76).

In his analysis of society, Marx argued that there are two fundamental components of a society: the base and the superstructure. The base comprises the forces of production and the social relationships of production, that is, the economy and class relations. It is the foundation on which a superstructure of social institutions is built, including the family, the education system, ideas and beliefs (what Marx calls 'ideologies'), the law and the political system. The base thus determines all other relationships and institutions in society: in Western society, the capitalist economic system and, central to this, the unequal class structure, are supported and maintained by all other institutions in society. People are encouraged to hold ideas and values which support the status quo: through socialisation they are indoctrinated into a 'false consciousness' which allows them to accept their subordination. Macionis and Plummer call this 'capitalist common sense' (1997: 78). But Marx was not pessimistic about the possibility of change. On the contrary, he believed that class conflict was inevitable, and that industrial capitalism laid wide open the contradictions and inequalities inherent in the capitalist system. Because of this, capitalism held within it the seeds of its own destruction; as 'class consciousness' developed, so the proletariat would rise up and overthrow capitalism (Marx and Engels 1976).

Marxist approaches have been criticised for being too simplistic and too mechanistic; underestimating the importance of ideology as a force in its own right and ignoring the importance of other inequalities such as those of 'race' or gender. Fulcher and Scott record that Marx himself was led to say 'I am not a Marxist', because he was unhappy about the claims being made in his name (1999: 32). Conflict theories and critical perspectives in sociology both developed as a challenge to what has been called 'crude' Marxism, taking on board some of the lessons of the interpretive paradigm while drawing on a Marxist analysis of structure. Ralf Dahrendorf (1957), for example, explored conflict from the standpoint of the unequal distribution of 'authority': those in power have a vested interest in holding on to their privileges; those who are ruled have an interest in seeking to alter the distribution of power. Because of these differences, Dahrendorf argues, people tend to form into 'social classes' (see Fulcher and Scott 1999: 58).

Critical theorists have developed Marx's ideas much further. Marx himself believed that a critical, self-conscious approach was essential for understanding society and for changing it. Authors such as Antonio Gramsci writing in the 1920s were pioneers of the development of a form of Marxist thought that broke with earlier, dogmatic versions of Marxism. Although little known in his day, Gramsci had a huge impact on radical thinking in the 1960s and 1970s (Fulcher and Scott 1999: 59). Gramsci (1971) criticised Marxism's insistence that ideology is subordinate to, and subsumed by, the economic system. He argued instead that ideology has power in its own right and that individuals must be led to socialism through ideology. Gramsci's ideas are closely connected with those of the 'Frankfurt school' (Max Horkheimer, Theodor Adorno and Herbert Marcuse) initiated in 1923. Sociologists from the Frankfurt school were critical of both capitalism and Soviet communism, and at the same time emphasised the importance of an exploration of psychic and cultural processes in order to understand society (Marsh *et al.* 1996: 91). Another critical theorist, Jurgen Habermas (1981a and b), has been highly influential in arguing that both structural and interactionist approaches are necessary; that neither alone provides a satisfactory base for social theory. He argues that only an interest in 'emancipation' (what he calls 'critical-dialectical thought') can liberate people from ideology and error, and bring about the self-determination and autonomy that was Marx's ultimate goal of human history (Fulcher and Scott 1999: 60).

Critical writing has developed greatly in recent years, moving beyond class-based explanations and taking on board lessons from both feminism and the anti-apartheid and black[6] movements (see Harding 1987, Smith 1988, Hill Collins 1990, Hall 1991 and Davis 1997). This writing continues to assert that knowledge is structured by existing sets of social relations and that these sets of social relations are oppressive in nature. But now, instead of proposing that class is the main centre of oppression, analysis also explores other forms of oppression including most frequently class, gender and 'race' (for example, Harvey 1990).

The interpretive paradigm

The interpretive paradigm offers a very different way of conceptualising society to that proposed by structural approaches of functionalism or Marxist perspectives. The interpretive or 'action' perspective no longer assumes that the whole of society is a unitary social system. Instead the focus is on the small-scale interactions between individuals and groups within society, and the ways in which meanings and definitions are constructed in particular ways at particular times. Interpretive or interactionist approaches are interested, therefore, in interrogating individuals to find out why they behave in a certain way and in investigating the areas of ambiguity and negotiation which are central to our actions and thought processes.

Max Weber is an early exponent of interpretive perspectives in sociology. Like Durkheim and Marx, Weber was involved in attempting to understand and explain the changes that were taking place in the development of a new industrial society. And in common with Marx, Weber believed that the essence of capitalism is the pursuit of profit. But Weber was critical of what he saw as Marx's over-emphasis on economic or material explanations for historical development. In his study of religion (first published in 1902), Weber argues that the Protestant religion, infused with values which supported and encouraged capitalist thinking, influenced economic behaviour, not vice-versa (Weber 1974). For Weber, it was rationality that was the driving force behind capitalism: modernity was to be understood as 'the triumph of rationality over all other forms of action' (Bilton *et al*. 1996: 89). The major problem for modern industrial society was not, then, economic inequality but 'the stifling regulation and dehumanisation that comes with expanding bureaucracy', leading to what Weber calls an increasing 'disenchantment with the world' (Macionis and Plummer 1997: 87). Weber was not, however, interested in analysis only at the macro-level. He argued that sociology had to start not from structures, but from people's actions (Fulcher and Scott 1999: 40). Individuals are creative actors whose actions determine both present society and the course of history. This does not imply that there are no constraints on individuals: constraints do exist, but what is significant is how people perceive those constraints. Weber emphasised the importance of understanding the subjective meaning that every 'actor' brings to a social situation: each social situation is established and sustained by the meaning brought into it by participants. It is this unique ability of human beings to interpret the world around them and choose to act which Weber sees as the key concern of sociology. Sociology should seek to understand ('verstehen') the theories of actors themselves rather than constructing expert theories of social systems (Bilton *et al*. 1996: 88). The principal concepts used by social scientists (e.g. capitalism, bureaucracy, the nation state) are, for Weber, no more than 'ideal types' – they are analytical devices constructed by social scientists to make sense of the world (Fulcher and Scott 1999: 42). This does not suggest that they have no meaning or worth. If constructed well, with large enough sample sizes, they can be useful tools. But, Weber warns, they will always be from one-sided, value-relevant standpoints; there are no universal truths valid for all time.

Weber's insights have been hugely influential in the development of later feminist and postmodern perspectives in sociology. In addition, the interpretive tradition in sociology, building from the work of Weber, has sought to understand the social context of human behaviour. Although there are a number of theoretical perspectives which can be described as interpretive sociology, the best known of these are *symbolic interactionism*, *phenomenology* and *ethnomethodology*.

Symbolic interactionism grew up in the 1920s and 1930s in the work of American sociologists including William Thomas, Charles Cooley and George Herbert Mead (1891–1939). Symbolic interactionism emphasises the flexibility of individual responses to social situations; its central concept is meaning and the variability of meaning in everyday life. George Herbert Mead (1934), for example, emphasised that 'the self' is a social construct, and that the way that individuals act and see themselves is in part a consequence of the way other people see and react to them (Muncie and Fitzgerald 1981: 412). In this way, individuals learn to behave differently in different situations. Erving Goffman (1922–1982) developed this further, describing social interaction as a form of theatre, in which we all play out roles in the drama of life (Goffman 1969).

Phenomenological approaches, originating in the ideas of Husserl and Schutz in the 1920s and 1930s, and later developed by Berger and Luckman (1967), investigate the ways in which the everyday world comes to be seen as normal, 'natural' and taken-for-granted. We are born into a preconstructed social world which has both objective and subjective meaning – it becomes a 'thing' whenever we name it and treat is as such (see Fulcher and Scott 1999: 56). Thus something like 'the family' appears to be separate from us as family members.

Ethnomethodology, while continuing to accept that individuals construct their social world, is particularly concerned with the underlying rules which govern everyday behaviour (Garfinkel 1967). Garfinkel is interested in how people account for their actions and interactions: what they choose to leave in, and what they choose to omit. There is no such thing, he argues, as a complete story: we cannot understand action and interaction until we know the context, the background, the knowledge and assumptions that underpin it. Bilton explains this as follows: 'Whereas symbolic interactionism focuses on the importance of verstehen ... ethnomethodology attempts to show how verstehen works' (Bilton *et al.* 1996: 93).

Interactionists of all perspectives have been criticised for failing to take account of the reality of power in society. Because groups and individuals have differential access to the process of creating meaning in a situation, explanations which are based on meaning may lose sight of the broader issues of power and inequality. Nevertheless, they have proved a powerful corrective to the determinism of large-scale structural theories.

Feminist perspectives

From the 1970s onwards, feminism has acted as a commentary on, and corrective to 'malestream' (masculinist) sociology, contributing to the development of sociological knowledge while at the same time challenging and confronting the ways in which that knowledge is created and recreated. Feminists have drawn attention to andro (male) centred language and practices in conventional sociology and explored what a feminist sociology might look like. For some feminists this has meant building a sociology which is apart from conventional sociology, centred on women's experience and a feminist standpoint (Harding 1987, Smith 1988). For others the task of feminist sociology has been to gender the social: to work within and beyond sociology to explain and to understand gender relations at the same time as extending the parameters of sociology into new areas, including housework (Oakley 1974), sexuality and heterosexism (Lees 1986), violence against women (Dobash and Dobash 1979). This work has effectively transformed a sociology which was previously mainly concerned with 'public' issues to one which now recognises the existence of 'private' issues (Maynard 1990).

Feminism is, of course, not one single ideology or one simple movement. There are as many feminisms as there are sociologies, so that we can find proponents of liberal, Marxist, socialist, radical, psychoanalytic, postmodernist, post-structural and black feminism. Within each broad grouping there are significant differences in approach and orientation, as well as areas of overlap and agreement. Some feminist approaches share with Marxist approaches their insistence on the impact of overriding structures in society, both economic and patriarchal. While Marxist feminists accept the dual importance of class and gender in society, radical feminists have argued that patriarchal structures have central power to determine the nature of women's experience in society. Other feminist perspectives are more interested in developing understanding of individual action and meaning (an interpretive approach) rather than taking on board large-scale 'grand' theory. What does unite feminists is a shared experience of gender oppression and a will to change this. Kelly, Burton and Regan propose: 'Feminism for us is both a theory and practice, a framework which informs our lives. Its purpose is to understand women's oppression in order that we might end it' (1994: 28).

Feminist sociologists in recent years have been confronted with a growing recognition that some of the building blocks of the feminist enterprise do not seem to be on as solid a foundation as they did in the early days of the Women's Movement. Black women, gay women and disabled women have all pointed out that a single category 'woman' is not tenable; that white middle-class women may have more in common with white middle-class men than do middle-class women and working-class women (see Fulcher and Scott 1999: 65). This does not, however, mean that gender oppression has disappeared. On the contrary, women's lives continue to be structured by oppression based on gender.

Black perspectives

Just as women have highlighted the implicit sexism in conventional sociology, so black women and men have drawn attention to the racist assumptions which are rooted in sociology. Not only has sociology largely disregarded a large proportion of the world's population in the so-called Third or Developing World, it has also, along with feminism, tended to ignore the experience of indigenous black people living in Britain and in the United States (Maynard 1990). This is not, however, to lose sight of the reality that there is wide diversity between and within black cultural and ethnic groups. Maynard explains her use of the term 'black':

> The term 'black' is not meant to refer to a fixed cultural identity
> ... It is a political label which acknowledges that the political,
> social and ideological force of racism creates a gulf between white
> people and those whom they oppress, on both a face to face and an
> institutional basis.
>
> (1990: 280)

Black and white sociologists have been concerned to explore the nature of 'race' and racism, as well as to explore the interconnectedness and uniqueness of different experiences and different forms of oppression. For black and white feminists, this has meant working to find ways of understanding the contradictory nature of women's oppression (Hill Collins 1990, Ramazanoglu 1989).

Postmodernism and post-structuralism

Postmodernist perspectives in sociology are prefaced by the assumption that the society in which we are living is qualitatively different from the society envisaged by the early sociological writers. Whereas early sociologists sought to describe and explain the conditions of 'modernism' (that is, industrial, urban, technical, scientific, bureaucratic, rational society), contemporary writers (for example, Bauman 1992, Kumar 1995, Parton 1996) conceptualise themselves as living in a 'postmodern' society, or at the very least an advanced form of 'modernism' in which the certainties of the old world have disappeared. Today's society is envisaged as a pluralistic, individualistic one, a 'multiplicity of voices'. There is a contingency about our being: everything is fluid and changing. We inhabit a host of different identities of class, 'race', ethnicity, gender, age, sexual orientation, and we may choose which identity we will forefront in different situations. And there is no single, 'true' theoretical perspective (no 'grand theory') which can explain and interpret our experience. The consequence is that life may feel fragmented and disparate: we do not always know whom we are and how to behave. This is a politics of 'difference', not of class or of gender (Hekman 1990, Weedon 1987).

Postmodern writers argue that there is no 'master identity' which determines everything else, just as there are no universal categories of experience and explanation and no 'grand narrative' of history as ever-unfolding progress and advancement. Mouzelis suggests with more than a hint of irony that 'given the fragile, chaotic, transient and discontinuous character of the social, any holistic theory imposes an order and a systemness on the social world that, in fact, exists only in the confused minds of social scientists' (1995: 42). Kumar offers a cautious overall assessment of postmodernist ideas: 'The contemporary world may not be simply or only postmodern; but postmodernity is now a significant, perhaps central, feature of its life, and an important way of thinking about it' (1995: 195).

There are a number of features which are said to be characteristic of postmodernity, including, crucially 'globalisation'. Fulcher and Scott (1999: 456–7) state that globalisation refers to the growing integration of societies across the world, through global organisation, global interdependence, global communication and global awareness. Globalisation brings with it scope for a greater understanding of the needs and problems of different cultures and societies throughout the world. It also, however, poses potential threats. As Bilton *et al.* explain, as transnational companies operate an increasingly sophisticated global market, so traditional customs and patterns of consumption and distribution can be undermined (1996: 75). Kumar takes a more optimistic view. He argues that globalisation can lead to particularisation and diversity, not just standardisation and uniformity, as globalisation's critics claim. This is because to continue to be successful in a world market, capitalism needs to diversify and individualise its products (1995: 189).

Post-structuralists, in common with postmodernist writers, reject the 'essentialism' of conventional sociological writing. While structuralists such as Saussure (1974) believed that the meaning which is produced in language is fixed, post-structuralists view meanings as multiple, unstable and changing (Featherstone and Fawcett 1995).

Michel Foucault (1926–1984) argues there is no such thing as set or objective meaning, but instead power, language and institutional practices come together in 'discourse' at specific moments in time to produce particular ways of thinking (Foucault 1977). Discourse is for Foucault more than simply verbal representation or even a way of thinking and producing meaning. Discourses are ways of regulating knowledge: 'practices that systematically form the objects of which they speak' (1972: 49).

Postmodern approaches have had a massive impact on the development of ideas, not just in sociology, but in literature, cultural studies and other disciplines (Fulcher and Scott 1999: 66). We can see postmodern ideas in increasing evidence in the social work literature of the 1990s. Howe (1994), Parton (1994) and Tuson (1996) have all used postmodern ideas to interrogate social work in general; Parton, Thorpe and Wattam (1997) have taken this into a specific exploration of child abuse/child protection; I myself have drawn directly on a Foucauldian framework in my historical analysis of the development of social work (Cree 1995). What these accounts share is an acceptance that social work is a creature of 'modernity': that it grew up alongside the social sciences as a means of explaining and improving the human condition. Social work theory and practice today are presented as fragmented and unclear, demonstrating all the uncertainties and ambiguities of postmodern life. Postmodern approaches have not, however, been without their critics. Postmodern perspectives have been severely criticised for lacking an adequate analysis of power and for a relativism that encourages pessimism and despair. Smith and White (1997) argue that a postmodern analysis in social work is 'ethically flawed'. They continue:

> In minimising the continued role of the state, and in collapsing all ideology and subjectivity into discourse, the often grim, lived realities of oppressed groups may be reduced to 'difference' and, in the process, pressing (emancipatory) social imperatives may become obscured.
>
> (1997: 293–4)

Looking ahead

I would like to finish this chapter by restating the reasons why a sociological approach is both helpful and necessary in social work. I will also locate myself within the sociological tradition, setting out my own position in terms of the sociological perspectives discussed in the chapter and in the book as a whole. The chapter ends with a Practice Example that is designed to illuminate the distinctiveness of a sociological approach to an everyday social work task.

Research into service-users' views of social work practice has consistently highlighted that effective practice depends on the combination of good interpersonal skills and clear, systematic, organised practice (Fischer 1978, Rees 1978). In a review of evaluative research on social work, Sheldon (1986) has argued that, when social work activities are clearly focused, problems clearly identified and specified goals set with service users, then studies produce positive results. Howe (1987: 7) argues that to achieve such structured practice, social workers must ask the following questions in every situation:

• What is the matter?
• What is going on?
• What is to be done?
• How is it to be done?
• Has it been done?

At each of the above points, a theoretical approach will be employed, explicit or otherwise. Social work practitioners at times seem to wish to deny the relevance of theory: there is a popular anti-intellectualism in contemporary social work practice (Hardiker and Barker 1981). Yet everything we do and believe is rooted in one theoretical approach or another. Reflective practitioners are aware that different theoretical positions produce different sets of questions and different answers. It is vital, therefore, that we bring a critical mind to our work; that we consider carefully the questions and answers that underpin our practice. Bauman asserts that sociology 'defamiliarizes' things: it takes us away from our comfortable, common-sense views and makes us more sensitive to the ways that these opinions are formed and maintained (Bauman 1990). Four further questions must therefore be addressed of each theoretical perspective (list adapted from Young 1981):

• What view of human nature is assumed?
• What view of society and social order is assumed?
• What are the implications of holding such a position, for individuals, their families, friends, communities and for society? are they positive or negative, and for whom?
• How does this theoretical perspective fit with what is already known from other reading and research or from personal experience?

All these questions are central to social work practice, as they are to our reading and understanding of the concepts and issues explored in this book.

My own perspective is best described as critical postmodern, in that it brings together insights from both critical and postmodern perspectives. In keeping with a critical tradition, I accept the importance of analysing individuals within wider social structures and systems of power relationships, particularly those of class, 'race', gender, age and disability. At the same time, however, I value the interpretive position because of its insistence on the centrality of human agency – the capacity which individuals have to bring choice and meaning to their lives. Moreover, I find postmodern approaches make sense of the world in which we are living and feel encouraged by the possibilities which postmodern analysis offers: if all things are contingent, then resistance and change may indeed be possible. (For a fuller discussion of the usefulness of making connections between postmodern and critical theory in social work, see Leonard 1997 and Pease and Fook 1999.)

Sociological perspectives: a practice example

You have been asked to carry out an initial investigation on a fourteen-year-old white boy who has been truanting from school and has recently been apprehended trying to sell car radios.

A psychological approach might be to look at the boy himself: his age and stage, his family relationships, his early childhood experiences, his psychological needs, his relationships with siblings and peers.

In contrast, a sociological approach would concentrate on the larger questions, about the structural place of young white men in society: about masculinities, about class and structural disadvantage, about education and youth unemployment, about the construction of 'whiteness', about the organisation of white working-class families and communities, about poverty, marginalisation and inequality. Sociologists may also ask why young people have been targeted for special scrutiny and condemnation as 'dangerous' in society, and why the behaviour of working-class youth (and that of black youth in particular) is treated significantly differently to that of white middle-class youth. Finally, they may wish to examine the context of late twentieth-century consumerism and New Right values of individualism and individual property.

Recommended reading

- Bauman, Z. (1990) *Thinking Sociologically*, Oxford: Basil Blackwell (an easy to read, stimulating text).
- Mills, C.W. (1959) *The Sociological Imagination*, Oxford: Oxford University Press (this is a classic text, well worth a read, in spite of the passage of time).

There are also a number of very large sociology handbooks geared mainly at undergraduate sociology students. I would strongly advise potential buyers to look at these in a bookshop or library and choose the one that the reader finds most accessible in terms of structure and language. Four recently published handbooks are:

- Bilton, T., Bonnett, K., Jones, P., Skinner, D., Stanworth, M. and Webster, A. (1996) *Introducing Sociology*, Third edition, Basingstoke: Macmillan.
- Fulcher, J. and Scott, J. (1999) *Sociology*, Oxford: Oxford University Press.
- Macionis, J.J. and Plummer, K. (1997) *Sociology: A Global Introduction*, New Jersey: Prentice Hall.
- Marsh, I., Keating, M., Eyre, A., Campbell, R. and McKenzie, J. (1996) *Making Sense of Society: An Introduction to Sociology*, Harlow, Essex: Addison Wesley Longman.

2 Family

Introduction

The family occupies a central position in social work theory and practice across the whole range of social work sectors, not only in children and families' work but also in community care and criminal justice. Much of what we think and do as social workers is underpinned by what may be unchallenged, unrecognised assumptions about the nature of the family and its relation to society. It is important, therefore, to look critically at the family and at our ideas and beliefs about the family so that social work policy and practice can reflect a deeper understanding of the contradictions and complexities which characterise both family life and the relationship between the family and the state.

This chapter is organised in three sections. In the first section, I will consider what we mean by 'family', clarifying the differences between family, household and kinship structures, and identifying the persuasive nature of familial ideas and practices. The second section goes on to examine historical, cross-cultural and sociological approaches to the study of the family. The final section will look at families in the UK in the 1990s, giving attention to the diversity of family arrangements.

Definitions

Why define the family? After all, we have all grown up in a family, of one kind or another. But that is the point: *of one kind or another.* Conventional wisdom (as well as much sociological writing) seems to suggest that 'the family' is one entity or institution; that 'the family' can be equated with the 'nuclear family' of husband, dependent wife and children. This is the assumed norm of much advertising, housing and social policy: the 'cereal packet norm family' of husband at work, happy smiling wife at home and two children, most often presented as a boy and a girl (Leach 1967). Yet we know that there are a host of families that do not fit this 'ideal', most obviously, lone parent families and dual income partnerships. Abbott and Wallace point out that the stereotypical nuclear family is in fact quite rare. Only one in twenty households in Britain at any one time conforms to this stereotype (1990: 73).

But here the confusion arises. I have slipped from talking about the family, to talking about the household, and the two are clearly not synonymous. Drawing on the work of Ball (1974), Muncie and Sapsford suggest a way of distinguishing between the family and the household (1995: 10). The family is presented as a group of people bound together by blood and marriage ties, but not necessarily located in one geographical place. The household, in contrast, is a spatial category where a group of people (or one person) is bound to a particular place. This characterisation is useful in that it encompasses those families who are living apart, or whose children have left home or gone to boarding school.[1] But there are problems with it too. While the distinction between family and household may work as a factual statement, it may not fit how people feel about who is in their family – for example, people who live together who are not married (with or without children) or lone parents with an adopted child or children. It is also possible that a person living alone, perhaps with a pet to care for, may see her/himself as part of a family.

Giddens defines the family as 'a group of people directly linked by kin connection, where the adult members take responsibility for caring for children' (1989: 384). But what about families that do not have children? And what is the special significance of 'kin connection' or the concept of kinship more generally? Studies of kinship demonstrate that there are many historical and cultural differences in expectations of kinship and parental responsibilities (Allan 1996). It is not difficult to identify those who are related to us: our aunts and uncles, brothers and sisters, parents and grandparents, cousins, nephews and nieces, in-laws, second cousins, etc. (our 'kin set'). But the list might be large or small, and it tells us nothing about either the quality of kin relationships or the variability of kin obligations. Finch and Mason's (1993) study of kin relationships and responsibilities finds support for the supposition that kin relationships are a significant source of assistance for many people. But their study also makes it clear (as will be discussed more fully in Chapter 6) that kinship commitments cannot be guaranteed automatically. Rather, they are built up over time in the context of relationships between people and are the subject of negotiation and compromise (1993: 169).

Family ideology

'The family' is, of course, more than simply a practical living arrangement or a grouping focused on the upbringing of children. It is a social institution, steeped in all the beliefs (religious, secular, intellectual and moral) which any one society at a given moment has about the family: what it is and what it should be. Debates about the family are therefore never neutral: when sociologists (such as Morgan 1995) bemoan the breakdown of the family, or when politicians declare themselves to be 'the party of the family' (as both Labour and Conservative governments in the UK have done), it is the 'traditional', nuclear family which they are talking about. All other types of family are defined with reference to the nuclear family (Muncie *et al.* 1995: 10). The term, 'the family', thus carries with it a collection of very specific meanings and assumptions about men and women, about children, about work, about sexual behaviour and about caring. Drawing on Beechey (1986), family or familial ideology (also called 'familism') makes three inter-connected claims:

1   The co-resident, conjugal, nuclear family is universal, normal and desirable;
2   The sexual division of labour is universal, normal and desirable;
3   Heterosexuality is universal, normal, and desirable.

Family ideology is, however, not just a set of beliefs about the nuclear family. It is also demonstrated (and institutionalised) in a range of practices which uphold and promote that specific view of family life. Social policies and the welfare state as a whole are built on the assumption that the nuclear family is the best arena for raising children and good for society as a whole (see, for example, Barrett and McIntosh 1982). In addition, it has been argued that social work practice is itself structured around an outmoded, patriarchal, white and middle-class concept of family life (see Brook and Davis 1985, Wilson 1977). (The relationship between social work and the family will be explored later in the chapter.)

In summary, in embarking on a study of the family, we must be aware exactly what is under discussion: is it the nuclear family or families in all their diversities? Is it families or households? Historical, cross-cultural and sociological studies have all played a part in building and sustaining knowledge and assumptions about the nuclear family in particular and families in general.

Historical accounts of families and social change

Much of what we know about social change in families has its origins in the writings of historian Philippe Aries. Aries' (1962) account of the differences between the medieval family and the industrial family set the tone for much of the historical and sociological analysis of the development of the 'modern'[2] family. Aries depicted the medieval family household as a stable economic unit in which three or more generations of one family worked and lived together, alongside various apprentices, lodgers and servants, and other unrelated adults. There was, he maintained, little notion of private space as something to be valued or sought after, and scant evidence of love and affection between either husbands and wives or parents and children. Aries contended that industrialisation and urbanisation broke down the extended family household unit and put in its place the 'modern' family, that is, small-scale, intimate, child-centred family units in which home and work became separate from one another, and geographical mobility commonplace.

Laslett (1972) challenges Aries' portrayal of medieval families, arguing that households in Britain have generally consisted of nuclear, not extended families. He studied parish records of 100 English country villages from 1564 to 1821 and found that the large extended family households popularised by Aries had never been common, because of late marriage and shorter lives. He identified that the mean household size in England (including servants) remained more or less constant at about 4.75 from the sixteenth century right through the industrialisation period until the end of the nineteenth century, when a steady decline set in to a figure of about 3.00 in contemporary censuses. This suggests that although the English family did get smaller, industrialisation could not be held to be the simple explanation for this. More than this, Laslett's research indicates that most people did not live in households made up of three or even four generations, as Aries had suggested. Instead, they lived in one or two generation families.

Young and Willmott's famous study of Bethnal Green in East London also serves as a corrective to Aries' analysis, finding that the extended family was 'alive and well' in the 1950s (Fulcher and Scott 1999: 356). Young and Willmott (1957) identified the resilience of kinship patterns in spite of geographical relocation. Working-class people still lived in close proximity to extended family members, and saw each other frequently. Their later study (1975) reports on the continuing social changes that were taking place throughout the

1960s. Married couples were now more likely to set up home together independent of their parents, and often at a geographical distance from them. As a result, couples were forced to rely on each other more, and to build shared friendships in place of the segregated activities and friendships of the past. Women (including those with children) were more likely to be working outside the home, while at the same time men were experiencing periods of unemployment. Young and Willmott suggested optimistically that these changes might be leading to the development of a 'symmetrical family', with more egalitarian and democratic relationships between husbands and wives, and both partners contributing to decision-making and financial resources.

Hareven (1996) challenges another myth about the medieval versus the modern family. She points out that there was widespread geographical mobility in pre-industrial societies. Far from inhibiting the extended family arrangement, industrialisation in practice led to an increase in co-residence, as incoming migrants to cities and towns lived with relatives at least in the initial settling-in stages. Hareven argues that most of the migration to industrial centres was carried out under the auspices of kin; villagers 'spearheaded migration for other relatives' by locating housing and jobs for them. In this way, migration often strengthened family and kinship ties by developing new functions for kin in response to the changing economic and employment conditions (1996: 24).[3]

Anderson (1983), in a seminal essay in which he explores 'what is new about the modern family', writes:

> however hard we look, the stable community in which most of the population grew up and grew old together, living out their whole lives in one place, seems to have been very rare in most if not all of non-Highland Britain at least since medieval times.
>
> (1983: 68)

He asserts that, contrary to popular view, it was in the twentieth century that rent restriction, council housing and a fall in population growth-rate produced in many areas more stable communities than had probably been found for hundreds of years. Although migration in the past may have been over a relatively short distance, lack of communication and transport systems suggest that the possibility of keeping in touch today is 'at least as good as in the past' (1983: 69).

In reviewing the historical evidence, Anderson concludes that many of the features that we think of as 'new' are a feature of the post-1945 period, rather than a product of industrialisation. Because of this, they do not necessarily tell us about families in the longer past. Three examples illustrate this well: family stability, the care for older people and family size.

Family stability

Anderson (1983) argues that it has not been proved that families were more stable in the past, since death did in the past what divorce does today in terms of family break-up, loss and separation. Historical studies demonstrate vividly that family life before the middle of the twentieth century was at least as disrupted as it is today. Families in the past suffered great disturbance: women dying in childbirth, men and women dying at an early age, high levels of infant and child mortality, men working away from home for months or years at a time in the armed forces, the merchant navy, or working as labourers building roads, railways and bridges far from home, children going into factory work or living-in service positions. Even into the twentieth century, two World Wars meant that families were often headed by lone parents or were re-formed or step-families.

Care for older people

Anderson (1983) also suggests that there is no evidence that families cared better for their older members in the past. Finch's (1989) historical investigation of family obligations explores in depth the idea that the family of the past was characterised by greater family loyalties and stronger family ties. She points out that there has been little change in patterns of co-residence for older people. Most married older people lived only with their spouses, and small but fairly constant proportions have always lived in residential institutions of one kind or another. Some older people have also chosen to live alone (then and now), and Finch warns against making an assumption that an older person living alone is somehow neglected, abandoned or uncared for by her or his kin. Wall's analysis of relationships between generations confirms this point. He argues that responsibility for older people in the past was commonly shared between the state, the family and 'other charitable minded individuals' (1992: 84). (See also Chapter 6 for a fuller discussion of family care.)

Family size and composition

This is not, however, to suggest that there has been no change in family size and composition. Social, economic and demographic changes have led to major changes in family size and composition. Households are much less likely to contain boarders, servants, apprentices and other unrelated individuals as well as parents and children. People are living longer and having fewer children. At the same time, the clustering of children into the earlier years of marriage has meant that the stage between the birth of the last child and the first grandchild has been much lengthened (Anderson 1983).

An alternative approach to family history

Hareven (1996) offers an alternative, dynamic way of conceptualising the family in history. She points out that studies which are based on one moment in time ('snapshot' studies) do not reflect the ways in which household structures change over time, so that one individual might live in many different family groupings over a lifetime. She is critical too of the implicit assumption that the family is a passive institution which is acted on by urbanisation, industrialisation or whatever. She argues instead that the family is an active agent, involved in planning, initiating and even at times resisting change (1996: 26).[4] She writes: 'Familial and industrial adaptation processes were not merely parallel but interrelated as a part of a personal and historical continuum' (1996: 30).

Cross-cultural studies

Cross-cultural studies have also contributed to the development of sociological and everyday notions about 'the family'. George P. Murdock, writing in 1949 (2nd edn 1965), examined the evidence from 250 societies throughout the world and claimed that:

> The nuclear family is a universal social grouping. Either as the sole prevailing form of the family or as the basic unit from which more complex familial forms are compounded, it exists as a distinct and strongly functional group in every known society.
>
> (1965: 2–3)

Murdock's research has been highly influential in providing evidence on which functionalist sociologists (such as Parsons 1951) have built their conceptual frameworks. However, a contemporary of Murdock, Reiss (1965), has challenged his findings by presenting his own investigations into some of the societies explored by Murdock. In reviewing

Murdock's work, he argues that, although societies which have nuclear families may be surprisingly common, that is quite different from demonstrating that this is always the case or necessarily the case (1965: 447). He concludes that what is universal about the family is not the nuclear family as such, but the raising of children. He writes: 'The family institution is a small kinship structured group with the key function of nurturant socialization of the newborn' (1965: 449).

Oakley's (1972) review of anthropological evidence on family and kinship systems confirms that there is widespread variation between societies in terms of family patterns and behaviour which is considered suitable for men and women. Most importantly, she asserts that men and women are not universally in all cultures divided into hunter-gatherers and carers of young children.

Contemporary cross-cultural (and within culture) studies support Oakley's findings. As we will explore in the last part of this chapter, there is widespread diversity of family arrangements and ways of organising roles within the family, even within the UK. For example, Abbott and Wallace (1990) point to families of Asian origin who continue to live in extended family groups, and West Indian families who are often assumed to be matrifocal (mother-headed). There are also many families in which people choose not to get married, or women with children work full-time, or men take the role of home-maker (1990: 83). There are, in addition, 'families of choice': strong, supportive networks of friends, lovers and even members of families of origin which 'provide the framework for the development of mutual care, responsibility and commitment for many self-identified non-heterosexuals (lesbians and gays, bisexuals, homosexuals, 'queers': the self-descriptions vary)' (Weeks, Heaphy and Donovan 1999: 111).

Gittins (1993: 8) asserts that there is no such thing as *the* family, only families. This is a good point to carry forward into our examination of sociological approaches to the family.

Sociological approaches to the family

The idea that the family is a key social institution has been central to sociology. However, sociologists propose very different definitions of the family, and these lead to equally different theoretical conclusions. Consensus approaches start with the assumption that there is one preferred, ideal family: the nuclear family. All other types of family arrangement are seen, to a degree, as problematic, non-functional and inadequate. Functionalist sociologists (and many politicians and news-paper columnists) look back to a 'golden age' of the family; to a time in the past when it is assumed that nuclear families predominated, when families 'looked after their own', when women and men 'knew their place'. In contrast, conflict approaches throw into sharp relief the services which the family provides for the state, and point out the potentially harmful aspects of family life for its members. Critical and postmodern approaches stress the diversity of family arrangements: extended families, restructured (re-formed) families, single (lone) parent families, 'families of choice' are assumed to be as valid and as 'normal' as conjugal (nuclear) families. In addition, using many of the arguments and evidence presented earlier, the notion that the nuclear family was ever the 'traditional', or 'normal' family set-up is challenged.

Functionalist perspectives

Functionalist perspectives on the family held sway in sociology between the 1940s and 1960s, and remain popular today, particularly in North American sociology. A functionalist approach, as outlined in Chapter 1, presupposes that social institutions develop to meet the needs of society; they play a positive part in maintaining the social equilibrium and harmony of that society. Functionalist writers are therefore concerned to identify the functions the family provides, and how these might benefit both family members and the wider society (Marsh *et al.* 1996: 412).

Parsons (1955) pioneered the functionalist approach to the family in the postwar period. He writes:

> The basic and irreducible functions of the family are two: the primary socialisation of children so that they can truly become members of the society into which they have been born; second, the stabilisation of the adult personalities of the population of the society.
>
> (1955: 15)

The significant word here is 'irreducible': without the nuclear family, children will not be adequately socialised to become members of society and the personalities of adults will not be 'stabilised'. In his later writing, Parsons (1951) argues that the sexual division of labour is central to the success of the nuclear family: there must be one primary wage-earner and one principal home-maker so that conflict and competition between men and women will be reduced. Work and family commitments are seen as separate and gendered: 'expressive' women and 'instrumental' men inhabit different spheres of domestic (private) and work (public) life; the specialisation which is at the root of domestic relationships thus mirrors the differentiation inherent in industrialisation. Just as important, a 'good marriage' for Parsons is one that includes children, since the functions as parents reinforce the functions in relation to one another as spouses (Parsons 1951, 1949).

The function of the nuclear family is not, however, understood only in relation to the well-being of individual family members. The nuclear family is also assumed to meet the needs of society. In setting out his analysis of social change, Parsons (1955) argues that the pre-industrial (extended) family had been a multi-functional unit that had met most of people's needs. Modernisation had brought with it institutional differentiation, as specialised institutions emerged to meet particular needs, and the family lost some of its former functions (see Fulcher and Scott 1999: 357–8). Parsons views this transformation positively, believing that the nuclear family form met the needs of the new, industrial economy for a mobile and adaptable workforce. He explains this in terms of the sexual division of labour: with only one 'breadwinner', and without an extended family to hold people back, important decisions about childcare and work could be made quickly and easily, without tension or conflict.

As Fulcher and Scott (1999: 358) observe, Parsons' approach has been much criticised for seeming to suggest that the patriarchal family with the gendered division of labour alone met the requirements of an industrial economy. Parsons did not give adequate attention to internal conflicts in the family, nor consider alternative ways of meeting the needs for socialisation and personality management, through different forms of family arrangement. Some critics have gone so far as to argue that the nuclear family exalted by Parsons was only ever visible in American middle-class families for a short time in the postwar period (Morgan 1975).

In spite of the critique, functionalist approaches have had an enduring place in the public and sociological imagination. In recent years, there has been much political, religious and media posturing (as well as sociological writing) about the presumed breakdown of the nuclear family, and about the 'evils' of lone parent families, divorce, working mothers, 'inadequate' parents and teenage mothers (see, for example, Morgan, 1995; Dennis and Erdos 1993). Allied to this, there have been concerns about the encroachment of 'the state' into the lives of individuals and families. It is suggested that there is increasing specialisation in the family, as outside agencies such as schools, health and social welfare agencies take over functions that used to be performed by the family. For some, outside intervention in family life is valued as a positive feature, propping up 'ailing families' and preventing others from getting into difficulty (Bilton *et al.* 1996: 488). For others, it is seen as a cause for concern: the state is perceived as becoming too involved in family life, thus leading to dependency amongst recipients of welfare services and an erosion of personal and parental responsibility. The solution for the current-day politician (whether New Right or 'ethical socialist' Left)[5] and the functionalist sociologist is a return to the 'traditional' nuclear family. This is evidenced in Margaret Thatcher's now famous assertion in 1987 that 'There is no such thing as society; there are only individuals and families' (cited in Muncie and Wetherell 1995: 62). It is also demonstrated by Davies *et al.* (1993), who call for a return to the 'stable nuclear family rooted in a coherent sexual ethic'. They write:

> The only institution which can provide the time, the attention, the love and the care ... is not just 'the family', but a stable two-parent mutually complementary nuclear family. The fewer of such families that we have, the less we will have of either freedom or stability.
>
> (1993: 7)

Such views, expressed both in Britain and in the United States,[6] have led to demands for the withdrawal of state benefits to lone mothers as the 'only way of re-establishing the traditional norms of married parenthood' (McIntosh 1996: 148). New agencies have also been created to reinforce the importance of families taking care of their own, for example the Child Support Agency, set up to enforce the payment of maintenance by absent parents to their families (Muncie and Sapsford 1995: 33). In addition, there have been changes in the organisation and delivery of health and welfare systems in the 1980s and 1990s in the UK, so that there is a greater stress on the role of the community, hence shifting responsibility back onto families, and often (but not exclusively) onto women in families. (This theme is picked up in Chapter 6.)

Marxist approaches

Although Marxist and functionalist perspectives both see the family as central to the operation of society, Marxist approaches present a very different set of understandings about the family. Where functionalists stress the benefits of the family for society, Marxist writers concentrate on the ways that the family perpetuates social inequality. The starting-point of a Marxist approach is that the family is ultimately dependent upon the dominant mode of production (here the capitalist economy) for its existence and form. As a consequence, dominant class interests have a central impact on family structure and functioning.

One of the earliest accounts of the development of the modern family was presented by Engels in 1884 in *The Origin of the Family, Private Property and the State* (Engels 1902). Drawing heavily on Marx's notes relating to the work of a Victorian anthropologist, Lewis Morgan, Engels argued that monogamous marriage and the nuclear family emerged because of the development of private ownership of property (see Bernardes 1997). Marriage enabled men to protect their inheritance, since through it they could ensure that their heirs would succeed them. The role of women was, in turn, a form of prostitution, since wives 'sold' their sexual and reproductive services and their fidelity in return for their material care by their husbands (Muncie and Sapsford 1995: 24). Engels believed that only a truly communist society where property and tasks were shared would guarantee the end of exploitation in the family (Marsh *et al.* 1996: 416).

Engels' analysis has been described as pioneering in its appreciation of the control of women's sexuality, but at the same time 'seriously flawed' in its conceptualisation of 'civilisation' (Muncie and Sapsford 1995: 24). Contemporary Marxist perspectives stress that the nuclear family services the interests of capital in three principal ways: by producing and reproducing labour power; by producing a site for the maintenance of a reserve army of labour; and by facilitating the consumption of vast quantities of consumer goods (Knuttila 1996: 271):

1   Production and reproduction of labour power: capitalism needs healthy, mobile workers for its production systems; it also needs class divisions to be reproduced. Labour power is produced and reproduced by the family, which provides workers with food and rest and at the same time socialises children into values which maintain the capitalist system and provide a refuge from, and counter-balance to the oppressions of the workplace. The family is, then, a 'haven in a heartless world' (Lasch 1977). The family in this way both encourages and maintains the capitalist system.

2   Reserve army of labour: women in the family have a special part to play, firstly, as suppliers of unpaid domestic labour at home, and secondly, as a reserve pool to be drawn into the workforce at times of labour shortage.

3   Unit of consumption: the family is an ideal unit of consumption for goods produced outside the home. Institutions such as the media sell us an image of family life and encourage greater consumption

in the family: consumer durables (from washing machines to lawn mowers to mobile phones) are sold to families as 'must-haves'.

As Knuttila accurately observes:

> If you are a producer of consumer commodities, what better system than one composed of hundreds of thousands of small-sized consumption units in the form of isolated nuclear families, which all compete with each other to have the latest and best of every possible household and personal consumer item?
>
> (1996 : 274)

This is not, to suggest, however, that Marxist accounts of the family have ignored the potential conflicts within the nuclear family system. Zaretsky (1976) argues that the pressure to create a refuge from capitalism places a heavy burden on family members, and particularly on women. He sees the housewife as a 'classic expression' of the contradiction in the family: 'her family's income may rise, technology may lessen the burden of work, but she remains oppressed because she remains isolated' (1976: 141). Sennett's (1980) account of the inevitable 'destructive gemeinschaft' in familial relationships provides further support to this analysis (see Chapter 5 for a fuller discussion of the term 'gemeinschaft').

In summary, there are clear connections between functionalist and Marxist analyses of the family. Both see the nuclear family as the product of the 'modern' age, sustaining and supporting the industrialised, urbanised way of life. Both also identify in the nuclear family a place of personal freedom and retreat from the pressures of the workplace. But where functionalists see the family in positive terms as supporting economic structures, Marxist accounts view the family as an instrument of class oppression. It is one institution among many which promote dominant societal values and perpetuate both structural inequalities and the exploitation of subordinate groups, such as women and children. This theme is developed in feminist analyses of the family.

Feminist approaches

Bernardes asserts that feminism has been the single most important phenomenon to influence family theorising (1997: 42). Feminist analyses of the family take up the issue of exploitation in the family: the family is conceptualised as an institution which oppresses women; it is therefore a locus of struggle (see also Nava 1983, Wilson 1977). Writing from a range of different feminist perspectives, feminists have brought to public attention a number of critical realities about family life, including domestic violence, rape within marriage, child sexual abuse, the sexual division of labour, housework and childcare issues. Underpinning the feminist critique of the family is the rejection of the functionalist notion that 'the family' is one unified interest group. Instead, feminists have pointed out that the family is 'a location where people with different activities and interests ... often come into conflict with one another' (Hartmann 1981: 368) and where relationships between family members are characterised by an unequal distribution of power, responsibilities and resources (Abbott and Wallace 1990).

Marxist and socialist feminists (for example, Beechey 1987, Smart and Smart 1978) have developed many of the arguments presented already, seeing the family as the central location of women's oppression. Barrett and McIntosh (1982) challenge what they see as the ahistorical nature of conventional Marxist accounts of the development of the family, and point out that nuclear family groupings existed before capitalism. They go on to analyse the impact of capitalism on women in the family, specifically examining the growth of the idea of 'the family wage' as a source of disadvantage to women. They argue that the 'family wage' idea benefited both capitalists and the organised male working class, and it gave men social and economic power in the home. Women, in contrast, have never been thought to be entitled to a 'family wage' for their work outside the family, thus justifying their low wages and at the same time restricting women's choices and reducing their economic power within marriage (Abbott and Wallace 1990: 79). More recent Marxist and socialist feminist analysis has explored the ways in which work outside the home has been restructured to take advantage of women's lower wages, again furthering women's oppression in the family (Beechey and Perkins 1987).

Radical feminist thinking explains women's subordination in terms of the relation between women and men, and emphasises men's power over women, instead of capitalist domination. Radical feminists point out that patriarchy (the domination of women by men) pre-dated capitalism, and so cannot be explained by the development of capitalism. The family, instead of being viewed as the glue which holds industrial capitalism together, is now seen as the principal institution which props up patriarchy (Delphy 1984, Delphy and Leonard 1992). It does so by securing personal domestic services for men, and by socialising girls and boys into gender-specific roles.

Some feminists have argued that the only way forward in the study of the family is to abandon altogether the concept of 'the family': in order to understand family life and the lives of women for the first time we must 'deconstruct' the family (Barrett and McIntosh 1982).

Others (for example, Bernard 1972, Stets 1988) have stressed that the best way forward for understanding the family is to look in detail at the experiences of family members, interrogating the feelings and relationships within families. (This is explored further in the section on Interpretive Approaches.) Some feminists have put feminist ideas into practice and have experimented with alternative family arrangements and collective households. One of the discoveries made by women involved in new collective households was that their lives changed little: they still found themselves largely responsible for childcare and housework duties, as Segal (1983) reveals in an entertaining depiction of life in a 1960s commune in London.

Fulcher and Scott (1999: 359) note that while the feminist critique of the family has been highly influential, explanations that rely on the concept of patriarchy have been strongly criticised. If patriarchy is universal, it must be assumed to be biological in origin. Marxist feminist writers such as Walby (1990) have rejected this biological determinism, and point out that the idea of patriarchy as a total system cannot explain the differences and changes that have taken place in gender relationships. Walby prefers to think in terms of patriarchal structures, and suggests that there are patriarchal structures other than the family, including trade unions and the state. Moreover, black writers have criticised white middle-class feminists for their lack of attention to differences within black families and the significance of the family for black and minority ethnic people living in a racist society (see Bhavnani and Coulson 1986). (This will be explored further, see pp.40–2.)

Interpretive approaches

In contrast to the broad view taken by much functionalist, Marxist and feminist writing, interpretive approaches to the family focus at the micro-level on the interactions between family members and on the meaning which the family has for different members.

Phenomenologists such as Berger and Kellner have investigated the role played by marriage in the social construction of reality. For them, marriage 'serves as a protection against anomie for the individual' (1971: 23); it is a place where the relationships of adults in society may receive validation. The family, likewise, is the place where children learn to internalise what will become their everyday common sense. The centre of analysis here is the process of socialisation: the ways in which children come to acquire the symbols or meanings of their given culture.

Another micro-level approach, social exchange theory, although influential in the United States, has been largely ignored by sociologists in Britain. Exchange theory suggests that people are motivated by self-interest and act rationally, weighing up the rewards and costs of behaviour and actions (see, for example, Blau 1964). A decision to get married, to start a family and even to get divorced is viewed as a utilitarian decision; the persistence and endurance of the family is explained in terms of the family's appeal to self-interest. Some exchange theorists are also interested in the impact of negotiations and 'exchanges' at the level of social groups and organisations (see Klein and White 1996: 74–6). An exchange framework, working as it does from the assumption that human beings are autonomous, rational actors, takes no account of power differentials within families or of the impact of wider structural forces or ideologies on individuals. Nevertheless, key ideas within social work practice, notably the notion of 'client self-determination', fit within this conceptualisation of the importance of the individual actor, free to choose her or his course in life.

Radical psychiatrists, such as Laing writing in *Politics of the Family* (1976) and Cooper in *Death of the Family* (1971), adopt a more critical perspective. They explore the destructive nature of family relationships, uncovering the reality that the intensity of family relationships can be damaging: love may be used as an emotional weapon to manipulate and smother children and partners (Marsh *et al.* 1996: 420).

Feminist writers have also criticised early interactionist approaches for 'obscuring asymmetry in relations between women and men, and for encouraging a benign view of family life that ignores the capacity of men to impose their definitions of reality upon women' (Cheal 1991: 138). Feminist interactionists have therefore set out to explore family relationships from the inside. For example, in a renowned study, Bernard (1972) discovered that within every marriage, there are two different relationships: 'his' marriage and 'her' marriage. (See also Stets' 1988 exploration of the interactive dynamics of control and domestic violence.)

Black perspectives

Black writers have drawn attention to much of the implicit racism in theorising on the family. Typically, sociological approaches to the family take as their norm the white, Eurocentric family (sometimes explicitly, but more frequently in an unspoken, unacknowledged way). White patterns of family organisation and white cultural and historical influences provide the setting for all discussions of the family. Black families, which may have very different forms of organisation, history and traditions, are treated as exceptions to that norm: incomplete and at odds with the white family, rather than of value in their own right. Elliot (1996) puts this in the context of the old 'host–immigrant' model of ethnic relations: the host society is viewed as culturally homogenous, while minority ethnic groups are depicted as immigrants, strangers, bearers of dangerous, alien culture.

Such inherent racism leads to inaccurate and incomplete theorising. On the one hand, it may encourage writers to stereotype both white and black families, seeming to suggest that there is only one white or one black family, ignoring the diversities of class and ethnicity. On the other hand, it may lead writers to miss the complexities of experiences of family life. For example, Marxist and feminist sociologists who have portrayed the family as an institution of oppression have failed to see that it may also be a primary avenue of support for family members living in a hostile, racist society. Bhavnani and Coulson (1986) take up this point:

> Whatever inequalities exist in such [black] households, they are clearly sites of support for their members. In saying this, we are recognising that black women may have significant issues to face within black households.
>
> (1986: 88)

In addition, Thorogood (1987) argues that the existence of Afro-Caribbean family structures (that are frequently female-headed, lone parent families) brings into question the usefulness of the concept of patriarchal domination. Put simply, 'a recognition of some black family structures, which are less likely to include a male breadwinner, leads us to question whether the family *per se* is *the* major site of black women's oppression, or whether such oppression more directly flows from their colonial and labour history' (Muncie and Sapsford 1995: 27). (See Bryan 1992, Dominelli 1997, and Gilroy 1992 for a critique of social work practice with black families.)

Black approaches to the family today take as their starting-point the differences between black people as well as their shared experience of oppression: differences of age, gender, ethnicity, culture, religion and class.[7] Class-based analyses of the family also encourage us to examine the ways in which the white nuclear family has been (and is today) supported and maintained by the labour of black people. Black working-class women work long hours as domestic servants caring for white children and doing housework for white families. While South Africa under the system of apartheid may have been a particularly extreme example of the practice of exploiting black women in the family, many white families in major cities of Europe and the United States are today maintained by the labour of black women. These women, while supporting white families (through their work as nannies, carers and cleaners) may at the same time be seen to be forced to neglect their own children in the process (Brittan and Maynard 1984, Graham 1991, and Gregson and Lowe 1994). (This is explored further in Chapter 6, alongside a critique by disabled feminists of feminism's lack of interest in disabled people's experiences.)

Family violence

A major theme to arise in the sociological and feminist literature on families has been the growing realisation that families, far from being 'a haven in a heartless world' (Lasch 1977), can be dangerous places. Sociologist Richard Gelles (1979) puts this graphically:

> The family is the most violent group in society with the exception of the police and the military. You are more likely to get killed, injured or physically attacked in your own home by someone you are related to than in any other social context.
>
> (quoted in Macionis and Plummer 1997: 487)

From the 1960s onwards, there has been an explosion of public and academic interest in violence against women (domestic violence) and violence against children (child abuse and particularly child sexual abuse). While there is not space in this chapter to do justice to the whole field of psychological, sociological and feminist approaches to family violence, I will, nonetheless, attempt to sketch the broad parameters of what has been a contentious and deeply challenging area of exploration.

Violence against women

Johnson (1995: 104) states that in the early 1970s, domestic violence became a political issue. What began in 1972 as a local campaign in Hounslow, London, against the elimination of free school milk led to the beginnings of the Women's Aid movement, and the establishment of a National Federation of groups and refuges for women throughout the UK. The perspective adopted by both the Women's Aid movement and by those researching domestic violence has been overwhelmingly feminist in orientation. It is argued that, because by far the greatest amount of domestic violence is perpetrated by men, and because a large part of *all* criminal violence is violence within the home by men against women, violence should be understood as a means through which men seek to control women; it is typical of a patriarchal society (Dobash and Dobash 1979).

Mullender (1996) in a review of what is known about domestic violence clearly demonstrates a feminist perspective. She asserts that both masculinity and male sexuality are socially constructed to be oppressive, so that men's abuse of women is 'an extension of normal, condoned behaviour in a context of social inequality, not individual deviancy ... Men wield power over women and all men benefit from this' (1996: 63). Domestic violence, she continues, 'is endemic and it is overtly or covertly sanctioned'. She concludes: 'We are not dealing with a few bad apples in the barrel but with the whole barrel' (1996: 64).

The feminist approach to domestic violence has not been without its critics. Some have challenged the focus on husbands' violence against wives, pointing out that women can also be violent in marital relationships (for example, see Straus and Gelles' 1986 study of marital violence in the United States). The findings from the Straus and Gelles study have proved highly controversial amongst feminist writers. Dobash and Dobash (1992) have stressed that women's violence against men is of a different order and scale to that of men's violence against women, and that women who are violent are usually defending themselves, rather than in the role of aggressor. Elliot (1996: 164) accepts this argument, but nevertheless points out that 'in a significant minority of relationships, only the woman is violent.' This is an area currently under investigation (for example, see Nazroo 1999).

Violence against children

It was in the 1960s in the United States and the 1970s in the UK, that child abuse (then called 'the battered baby syndrome') emerged as a social issue, soon to be followed by the discovery of child sexual abuse. Understandings of child abuse have been dominated by psychological, rather than sociological paradigms. There has been a huge investment of time and effort into identifying the characteristics of physically and sexually abused children as well as the profiles of abusers, both potential and realised (see Waterhouse 1997, Waterhouse, Dobash and Carnie 1994). Waterhouse (1997: 150) reports that explanations of physical abuse today tend to draw on 'complex models of the interrelationship between multiple factors', likely to include adversity such as inadequate housing and unemployment, poor parent–child relationships, factors in the child's personality, and poor parenting skills of parents. By comparison, explanations of child sexual abuse concentrate on the misuse of power by adults (mainly men) over children (most often girls) and have been influenced greatly by feminist perspectives. For example, in her study of sexual violence, Kelly (1988) explores the links between different forms of sexual violence (rape, child sexual abuse and domestic violence), and uncovers the similarities between the myths and stereotypes surrounding forms of sexual violence and the institutional responses to abused women and girls. She concludes that all these forms of sexual violence are rooted in one and the same thing, that is, in male power in a patriarchal society. She puts this strongly: 'Men's power over women in patriarchal societies results in men assuming rights of sexual access to and intimacy with women' (1988: 41).

Some feminist writers and other sociologists have been concerned about what they perceive as essentialism in the portrayal of men and women in studies of violence against children. The feminist historian, Linda Gordon (1988) raises this issue when she considers the case of women who abuse children. She writes:

> The role of women as child abusers is important because child abuse is the only form of family violence in which women's assaults are common. Studying child abuse thus affords an unusual opportunity to examine women's anger and violence. Unfortunately, feminist influence in anti-family-violence work has not historically supported such an examination, because of an ideological emphasis on women's peaceableness and a rejection of victim-blaming that have pervaded much of feminist thought.
>
> (1988: 173)

In summary, violence against women and violence against children have both alerted sociologists to what has been called the 'dark' side of family life. Families are evidently not always the safe havens that were imagined by functionalist sociologists. Feminist writers have contributed greatly to the development of understandings of family violence. The analysis is very much a continuing exercise within sociology and within feminism, as researchers and practitioners confront the realities not only of domestic violence and child abuse, but also in more recent years, elder abuse (see Phillipson and Biggs 1995). Within the violence literature today, issues of power and gender remain very much to the fore (see Fawcett *et al.* 1996). This leads us into postmodern and post-structural approaches.

Post-structuralist and postmodernist perspectives

Post-structuralist and postmodernist approaches to the family emphasise the instability of theories about the family. They argue that a grand theory of 'the family' is unworkable: instead new ideas emerge, become popular for a time and disappear; and theoretical frameworks have a tendency to break down when applied in particular contexts (Cheal 1991: 155). Postmodernism focuses on different kinds of families and on individualisation: on the individual adaptations and individualism that characterise some families accompanied by greater fluidity and different identities of sex and gender roles. Postmodernist writers also examine the contradictions within families, and the continuities as well as the changes, which have taken place.

Post-structuralist writers, in rejecting any monolithic ideas of 'the family', are concerned to understand the ways in which different discourses (knowledge, ideas and practices) come together at particular times in history to create and support particular ideas about 'the family'. Foucault (1977) argues that our understandings of the 'family' (its concept, its purpose and our expectations of it) are constituted by the very discourses which describe and explain it (Howe 1991: 153). In exploring the changing nature of discipline and power in society, Foucault (1977) identifies a shift in European societies, beginning in the seventeenth century, in the ways in which power was exercised over life ('biopower'), including sexuality. From then on, the control of citizens was no longer achieved by coercion or by the threat of the scaffold, but by new systems of classification and surveillance of social and specifically sexual behaviour. Central to this was the process of 'normalisation', that is, discipline through the family, the school and the community, watched over by new *social* professionals: social workers, health visitors, doctors, teachers, psychologists, armed with their new social science knowledge and practices. The new social experts held a dual function: their role was to treat at the same time as to define and judge the family (Howe 1991). Taking the argument further, Donzelot (1980) abhors what he sees as this 'policing of families'. He looks back to a patriarchal past where men were truly the heads of households and the state rarely intervened in family life. He contrasts this with the contemporary situation in which 'the family appears as though colonised' and there is now 'a patriarchy of the state' (1980: 103).[8]

The state, social work and the family

Developing a Foucauldian analysis, social work is without question part of the 'disciplinary mechanisms' of society: the expansion of social work has gone hand in hand with the increasing involvement of the state in surveying and controlling the lives of citizens. The purpose of social work's intervention in the family is to ensure the protection and well-being of children, while at the same time maintaining the legitimacy of the liberal state. Social work therefore can be understood as standing at a midway point between the individual and the state, between the private and the public spheres, acting as a bridge between the two. For Parton (1991), this is social work's 'crucial mediating role': it is social work which sets the standards of what constitutes 'normal family relationships' and what is 'good enough' parenting (1991: 214).

But if social work does set the standards of 'normal family relationships', as Parton suggests, in practice we can identify a great many different ways in which social work with the family has been organised, historically and in the present day. Historical accounts illustrate that there have been very different solutions to perceived problems in family life over the last 100 years or so. In the late nineteenth century in the UK, protecting children meant removing them from their poor families and transporting them to new lives overseas in Canada, Australia and New Zealand (see Colton *et al.* 1995). In the 1950s and 1960s, it meant placing deprived or illegitimate children for adoption with predominantly white, middle-class married couples (see Triseliotis 1980). But separating children from their parents of origin was not always the primary objective in childcare. Workhouses in England in the nineteenth century intentionally held onto children so that they could maintain contact with their parents.[9] Similarly, agencies such as Family Service Units and local authority Social Work (and Social Service) Departments have always struggled to keep so-called 'problem' families together. (For a fuller account of the historical development of social work with families, see Cree 1995, Holman 1988, and Parker *et al.* 1991.) Waterhouse (1997), in her analysis of changing standards of 'good enough' parenting, argues that social work's view of what is acceptable behaviour in the family is affected as much by public opinion as by its own internal, professional judgement. High public and professional tolerance reduces the numbers of children requiring investigation, registration and follow-up, low tolerance the reverse. Whatever benchmark is employed, she writes, 'universal standards for bringing up children and accepted limits of "good enough" parenting are likely over time to be affected' (1997: 149–50).

Current UK legislation evidences the complex and at times conflicting relationship between the state, social work and the family. The Children Act (1989) and the Children (Scotland) Act (1995) stress the importance of keeping families together, and set out their objective to strengthen parents' responsibility for their children.[10] However, both Acts also state that the welfare of the child must come first. This may inevitably lead social workers to take actions which effectively break up family units, by removing children thought to be at risk from home, or in the case of Scottish legislation, by prohibiting an allegedly abusive father from the family home (see Adams 1996, Hill and Aldgate 1996).

There is one last issue to be considered here. It has been contended that Donzelot and other writers influenced by Foucault have understated the significance of resistance in relation to surveillance and control in the social regulation of families. Dingwall *et al.* (1983, 2nd edn 1995) in their examination of child abuse argue that 'resistances' lie in both the culture and the structure of the social worker–client relationship. Social work encounters with clients are characterised by what they call 'the rule of optimism': an acceptance of parents' accounts and an acknowledgement that a charge of mistreatment is 'a matter of almost inconceivable gravity' (1995: 218). In addition, the structural constraints on social work agencies mean that they do not have the power of a family police force as envisaged by Donzelot. Dingwall *et al.* assert that, taken together, 'these restrictions constitute a powerful acknowledgement of the continuing force of family autonomy' (1995: 219). Two additional studies demonstrate that the relationship between social work and families is not a straightforward one of total imposition and restraint, but is instead marked by negotiation and at times resistance. See Gordon's (1988) research into women victims of family violence and care-giving agencies; and my own research, Cree (1995) into accounts of women using moral welfare agencies.

Summary

I have argued that, just as social work with families evidences its functionalist and modernist underpinnings, so it illustrates new ideas drawn from feminism, Marxism and anti-racist practice. Social work with families has changed as society has changed; there is no one family social work to be found everywhere, any more than there is one nuclear family. Postmodern perspectives suggest that the family as a living arrangement and as a social institution is constantly developing, as individuals negotiate and renegotiate their relationships and as society and other social institutions act upon and engage with the family in all its forms. Nevertheless, we must not lose sight of the importance of a structural, Marxist position. Adams (1996) argues that major changes in social and economic policies are needed if social workers are really going to be able to help families and reduce child abuse. He points to the worsening material conditions of many of the poorest families in the UK and suggests that, while systems approaches had the potential to point out that poverty and oppression was the issue, social workers have turned their backs on this, favouring instead narrow specialist therapeutic measures and 'risk' assessment. This is an important cautionary note to take into our examination of families in the UK in the late 1990s.

Implications for practice

We have reviewed a whole range of theoretical perspectives on the family, from macro-level functionalist and conflict approaches (Marxist and feminist) to micro-level interactive, and finally post-modern and post-structural conceptualisations. It is clear from the discussion that the social work task with families demon-strates its functionalist (and modernist) underpinnings. In function-alist terms, social work aims to socialise and if necessary, re-educate families into the norms and values of society. Its focus is not the social and moral education of *all* families (as is the pattern for the provision of health and educational services).[11] Rather, it is in the business of retraining and controlling society's casualties: those specific families who fall through the net of universalistic welfare. They may be 'problem families' (likely to be poor and socially disadvantaged, often lone parent families, often from minority ethnic groups) or they may be families whose members have already experienced family breakdown (such as families with foster children, adoptive families, etc.; see Adams 1996).

Since the 1980s, social work theory and practice with families has been under a sustained attack from a combination of academics, practitioners and researchers concerned to bring new Marxist, feminist and anti-racist understandings to social work. Some have focused their attention on social work theory, challenging traditional ideas and introducing in their place new feminist and anti-oppressive analyses (see Brook and Davis 1985). Some have been involved in researching social work practice, uncovering the durability of familial assumptions and stereotypical attitudes (see Langan and Day 1992, Maynard 1985). Others have devoted their energies to developing new models of practice, pioneering explicitly feminist, anti-racist, anti-discriminatory and anti-oppressive approaches to social work intervention (see Cavanagh and Cree 1996, Hanmer and Statham 1988, Perelberg and Miller 1990, Dominelli and McLeod 1989, Thompson 1997).

Feminist social workers and pro-feminist men in social work today are making a significant contribution to the development of theory and practice with men, women and children, seeking to build alliances with women and challenge conventional social work ideas about 'confidentiality' and 'professional expertise'. Mullender (1997) argues that women's problems are structural not individual: poverty, isolation, lack of access to work, relationships with violent partners, poor housing, being mothers of small children. The social work response to families must therefore reflect an understanding of wider sociological issues.

Changing families in the UK

There has been no shortage of statistical information on families in the UK in the 1990s. Censuses, government surveys, research studies and reports all contain different pieces of the jigsaw puzzle, presenting what at times can be a contradictory and confusing picture. Statistics are notoriously unreliable and open to manipulation (Huff 1973); one set of figures can appear to give quite different information, depending on how the statistics are set out and how they are contextualised. The 'family', as I have said, is the subject of intense negotiation and debate. In addition, research studies are always tainted in some way by the predispositions, values and beliefs of those who carry out and those who fund research (Gubrium and Silverman 1989). It is unsurprising, therefore, that it is impossible to step outside ideology to uncover pure 'facts' which are untainted by the theoretical perspectives and ideas which we have already explored. I will outline here the most pertinent changes which have taken place in families in the UK over the last thirty years or so. For further analysis, readers should refer to Marsh *et al*. (1996), Elliot (1996), the current issue of *Social Trends* and the *General Household Survey*. For changes affecting families in the United States, Rank and Kain (1995) offer a useful summary.

Changes in households

Demographic and social changes have led to a significant shift in patterns of households in Britain. A falling birth-rate, reduced infant and child mortality, a reduction in adult mortality and an increase in the number of very elderly people means that, although the average size of households has almost halved since the beginning of the twentieth century to 2.4 people per household in 1996–7, the number of households has been rising. There were in fact 7 million more households in Britain in 1996–7 than in 1961 (*Social Trends* 28, 1998: 42). This rise is largely connected to the striking increase in people living alone: the number of households made up of one person has doubled since 1961 (see Table 2.1). (Although the average household size in Northern Ireland is slightly larger at 2.8, the overall trends are the same as in the rest of the UK.)

Changes in one-person households

Women aged sixty years and over formed the largest proportion of people living alone in England and Wales in 1996. This proportion has been relatively stable over the last twenty-five years or so. In recent years, however, the largest increase in people living alone has been among men under the age of sixty-five years. This is seen as reflecting the decline in marriage and the rise in separation and divorce. It is projected that numbers of men living alone will increase further to form the largest type of one-person households within about ten years (*Social Trends* 28, 1998: 43).

Table 2.1 Households by type of household and family, Great Britain (percentages), 1961 to 1996–7

	1961	1971	1981	1991	1996–7
One person households					
Under pensionable age	4	6	8	11	13
Over pensionable age	7	12	14	16	15
Two or more unrelated adults	5	4	5	3	2
One family households					
Married/cohabiting couple with					
No children	26	27	26	28	28
1–2 dependent children	30	26	25	20	21
3 or more dependent children	8	9	6	5	5
Non-dependent children only	10	8	8	8	6
Lone parent with:					
Dependent children	2	3	5	6	7
Non-dependent children only	4	4	4	4	3
Two or more families	3	1	1	1	1
Number of households (=100%) (millions)	16.2	18.2	19.5	21.9	23.5

Source: Office of Population Censuses and Surveys; General Register Office (Scotland); General Register Office (Northern Ireland); Social Trends 28, 1998, Table 2.3: 42.

Changes in family composition

The proportion of 'traditional' households comprising a heterosexual couple with dependent children has fallen over the last thirty-five years to only 25 per cent of all households in Britain (31 per cent in Northern Ireland; see Social Trends 28, 1998: 42 and Table 2.1). There has also been a decline in so-called 'multi-family' households (where more than one family unit lives together), though it is acknowledged that this extended family pattern is still relatively common amongst some minority ethnic groups (Social Trends 28, 1998: 43). Changes in family composition mirror those affecting households. Families made up of married or cohabiting couples with dependent children have fallen, while lone parent families (particularly lone mothers with children) have increased almost three-fold from the 1970s to the 1990s. Most lone parents are women, reflecting the reality that children tend to stay with their mothers after divorce (*General Household Survey* 1998, *Social Trends* 28, 1998; see Table 2.2).

Changes in marriage and divorce

There has been a substantial decrease in first marriages in the UK since a peak in 1970. In 1995, there were 192,000 first marriages, which was half the number in 1970. In contrast, the number of divorces doubled over the same period. It is estimated that currently two out of every five marriages will end in divorce (*Social Trends* 28, 1998: 50).

Changes in conception and abortion

Parents today are choosing to have fewer children overall, and in recent

Table 2.2 Dependent children: by family type, Great Britain (percentages)

	1972	1981	1991–2	1995–6
Couples				
1 child	16	18	17	16
2 children	35	41	37	38
3 or more children	41	29	28	26
Lone mothers				
1 child	2	3	5	5
2 children	2	4	7	7
3 or more children	2	3	6	6
Lone fathers				
1 child	–	1	–	1
2 children	1	1	1	1
3 or more children	–	–	–	–
	100	100	100	100

Source: General Household Survey, Office for National Statistics, *Social Focus on Families* (1997), Chart 1.26: 24.

years women have been delaying having children or have chosen to remain childless. The average age of mothers for all live births was 28.6 years in 1996 in England and Wales (*Social Trends* 28, 1998: 53). Over one-third of all these births were outside marriage. Teenage conceptions in England and Wales have fallen slightly since a peak in 1991. Abortion figures, however, have continued to rise steadily over the last twenty years, so that in 1995, 20 per cent of all conceptions led to an abortion (*Social Trends* 28, 1998: 54). There has been a fall in the numbers of children available for adoption: 10,400 in 1981 and only 6,500 in 1996. Only 5 per cent of adoptions were of children under one year of age.

Continuity and change?

The statistics presented so far seem to confirm the notion that the family is in terminal decline and that the nuclear family is a thing of the past. However, a very different picture can be presented from the same sources. This suggests a changing but perhaps surprisingly resilient picture of family life, with continuity and change existing side by side, and a significant degree of geographical and cultural difference.

Social Trends reports that, in spite of the growth in lone parent families, most dependent children live in a family with two parents: four-fifths of all children (and an even higher proportion of South Asian children) in Britain lived in such families in 1996–7. (This figure has fallen, however, from nine-tenths of all children in 1970.) Not all of these families had married parents. Many more couples cohabit, either as an alternative to marriage, or in a period (often prolonged) before marriage. Nevertheless, nearly three-quarters of families headed by a person aged under sixty years were married couples, and the vast majority of these married couples had children (see Table 2.3). This finding is replicated in a recent research study of 6,000 mothers and fathers aged thirty-three years which found that approximately three-quarters of the sample group were living in first marriages (Ferri and Smith 1996).

There are major differences in types of household between different ethnic groups. Indian and Pakistani/ Bangladeshi households are more likely to contain dependent children and are less likely to be single-person households or to have experienced divorce than white families. At the same time they are much less likely to be headed by a lone parent than West Indian families (*Social Trends* 28, 1998). Most recent figures suggest that only three out of every ten Black Caribbean children are brought up by a married couple, compared with six out of ten black African children and eight out of ten white children. Nine out of ten Indian and Pakistani children are raised by married couples (Office for National Statistics 1996). Elliot (1996) outlines research centred on black families in Britain today. This research indicates that the Afro-Caribbean family pattern is distinctive in terms of the institutional weakness of marriage, the prevalence of woman-headed families, the marginality of men and the orientation of women to economic independence. Evidence from Asian families, in contrast, shows the reproduction of Asian ideas of family loyalty and obligation, the primacy of mothering in women's lives and of male authority (1996: 57).

Although we know that very many marriages end in divorce, many divorced people do go on to form new relationships and remarry. Figures suggest that around 15 per cent of lone mothers cease to be lone parents each year; it is estimated that on average lone mothers spend four years or less living alone (*Social Trends* 28, 1998: 45). Remarriages accounted for two-fifths of all marriages in the UK in 1995 (*Social Trends* 28, 1998: 50). In 1991, there were found to be half-a-million step-families, containing around 1 million dependent children (*Social Trends* 28, 1998: 51).

Statistics for births outside marriage similarly should not lead us to make easy conclusions about the demise of the family unit. Although there has been a significant rise in numbers of births outside marriage, figures for England and Wales suggest that in four-fifths of these cases, births were registered jointly by both parents; and three-quarters of these were parents living at the same address (*Social Trends* 28, 1998: 53).

In 1995, the British Social Attitudes Survey asked people about their attitudes to family and investigated how much emphasis was placed on family values. *Social Trends* (1998: 47) reports that most people were found to be family-centred, believing it important to maintain contact with close relatives and the extended family, even when they had little in common with their relatives.

Nevertheless, this is not to understate the changes which have taken place. Elliot (1996) identifies changes in marriage as particularly important in understanding changes in the family. The separation of sex from marriage, the reconstruction of marriage as a terminable arrangement, and the separation of childbearing and childrearing from marriage have all worked together to create widespread changes in the family and in the relationships between family members, and critically between fathers and their children. Changes that have taken place have, nevertheless, been accompanied by a large degree of ambiguity and uncertainty. Weeks (1986) describes the coexistence of 'traditional' and 'liberated' values and patterns of behaviour: the ideology of the family is so powerful, he argues, that in spite of the growing diversity of relationships and family groupings, there is little acceptance of this pluralism. Segal (1983, 1990) agrees with this assessment. She highlights the strong forces against change: the counter-revolutionary groups and pro-family movements which struggle to reinforce traditional family values (this connects with my earlier discussion about family ideology; see p.27).

Bernardes (1997) reminds us that, although it does seem likely that many families do pass through a stage in which there are two adults and one or two children, we should not therefore assume that they share a 'common experience'; there remains great variability in terms of wealth, 'race', culture, housing, work, etc., so that it is unlikely that families pass through essentially similar phases. There is also a structured differentiation within families, characterised by both the sexual division of labour and the lack of power of children within families.

Implications for practice

A careful examination of statistics suggests that as social workers we must hold onto the realities of families in *all* their forms:

- Families are distinctive, unique formations which carry very different meanings for individual family members and which undoubtedly change over time.
- Families are not inevitably either positive or negative: they have within them the capacity for support and security for family members, as well as the capacity for abuse and exploitation.
- The conjugal family continues to have widespread appeal: people today still marry and remarry in great numbers, whether by personal choice or through a system of 'arranged' marriage.
- Experience of family life is mediated by structures and institutions in society: by 'race', ethnicity, gender, age, sexual orientation, social class; by the law, the education system

and social policies; by dominant ideologies which are inherently conservative in orientation, as well as being sexist, racist, heterosexist and ageist.

• There has been an increasing unwillingness, particularly on the part of women, to accept the negative consequences of nuclear family life. New family arrangements (greater numbers of lone parents and more re-formed families) are the direct consequence of this. Gay men and lesbian women have also chosen to have children and to apply to adopt and foster children, thus challenging the boundary of what constitutes a family.[12]

Conclusion

Cannan (1992: 123) contends that it is not changing family structures which cause social problems, but the relationship between the family and the state, and policies and practices which the state implements to support or undermine certain family forms. This is a very important message to end with. We need to critically examine social work policies and interventions to consider where and when 'traditional' nuclear family arrangements are indeed being privileged over other family forms. We must be prepared to value other family patterns, and work with service-users to support them. Finally, we must hold to the fore the reality that there is no singular 'family perspective' or 'family needs'. On the contrary, members of a family are likely to have very different positions and perspectives, structured as they are by wider forces of oppression including gender, age, 'race', sexuality and disability.

Recommended reading

• Bernardes, J. (1997) *Family Studies: An Introduction*, London: Routledge (a readable book with strong opinions on the nuclear family).

• Elliot, F.R. (1996) *Gender, Family and Society*, Basingstoke: Macmillan (provides good theoretical material and an analysis of statistical data).

• Muncie, J., Wetherell, M., Dallos, R. and Cochrane, A. (1995) *Understanding the Family*, London: Sage (an edited collection with many interesting and highly relevant chapters).

3 Childhood

Introduction

It has been widely acknowledged that until the mid 1980s, there was surprisingly little sociological interest in childhood, either by classical sociologists or by North American sociologists (Qvortrup 1995). Where children appear in the main body of sociological writing, this is largely in the context of a wider investigation of something else, most frequently the family, the community or the educational system. Children emerge in the literature as adjuncts of their parents, their carers or their teachers, with little recognition that they might have a place of their own in sociological knowledge and enquiry. Sociological surveys and official statistics frequently did not consider even the presence of children in their data collection and analysis, further increasing their invisibility in sociological discourse (Qvortrup 1994).[1] The absence of an analysis of childhood in sociological writing is not only a historical phenomenon. Two recently published textbooks on sociology make no mention of childhood: children are again sidelined in discussions of education, childcare and changing family patterns (Bilton *et al.* 1996, Marsh *et al.* 1996).

The 'adultism' (Alanen 1994) in sociology has important consequences for sociology and for social work. Most importantly, the absence of children in sociological discourse presents a significant gap in knowledge and understanding of society. This can be likened to the historical position of women within sociology. Feminist sociologists have argued that traditional sociology is not simply sexist, it is flawed sociology; its knowledge base and its research practices lack validity because they have ignored or sidelined the experiences of women (Harding 1991, Stanley 1990). Feminist sociologists have struggled over the last twenty years to put women and women's experiences onto the sociological map: to challenge conventional 'malestream' sociology

and to build a new sociological theory and practice which has as its
core the experiences and 'standpoints' of women. Sociologists interested in children and childhood are similarly working today to make
sociology reflect the experiences and perspectives of children and
young people. The lack of a sociological analysis of childhood means that academic
and childcare discourse around childhood and children has been
created on the basis of ideas and models which are largely psychological in derivation. Much of what we understand about childhood is
rooted in psychological ideas about child development, adolescence
and socialisation, often described in functionalist, positivist language.
The individualising approach in psychology makes it difficult to see
that issues and difficulties faced by children and young people may be
structural in origin, located in the structural position of children as a
subordinated, marginalised group, rather than in individual personality or developmental stage (Saporiti 1994). More than this, Mayall
(1994) argues that psychological discourses which aim to classify,
divide up and control children may oppress children in practice.

The implications for social work are self-evident. Most of what
social work knows about childhood is informed by psychology: ask any
social work student what they can tell you about children and young
people and they will probably come up with notions about 'ages and
stages' or 'needs of children', demonstrating little awareness of the
partial and normalising nature of the frameworks they are using.
Similarly, dominant theoretical perspectives in social work with children tend to be individualistic in nature, seeking causes and
explanations in individual personality or family pathology rather than
in structural issues such as class, poverty or inequality.[2]

This chapter will examine two phases of sociological enquiry into
childhood: first, sociology's early (and continuing) interest in socialisation; and second, sociology's more recent concern with the
institutionalisation of childhood. Before going on consider sociological
approaches to childhood, it is necessary to set the parameters of the
discussion: to ask, what is childhood?

Definitions of childhood

The starting-point must be an attempt to define childhood – here our
difficulties begin. We can be fairly certain that childhood begins at
birth, or perhaps even at the end of infancy. But when does childhood
end and adulthood commence? By looking at this more closely, we
find that definitions and expectations of age groups are not fixed: they

change over time and among cultures, especially between rich and poor societies. Hence what we expect of children living in the streets of Brazil or India may be very different from our expectations of children in middle-class families living in suburban villas in the United Kingdom or France or the United States.

Legislation exemplifies this lack of clarity about childhood by failing to delineate the childhood/adulthood boundary in any precise way. This means that in the UK, there are different ages for marriage, for voting in elections, for having sexual intercourse, for driving a car, for buying cigarettes or alcohol, and for claiming social security benefits. Pilcher (1995) sets out the official ages of adulthood in modern Britain, as shown in Table 3.1.

Table 3.1 Official ages of adulthood in modern Britain

Age	Context
8	Age of criminal responsibility (Scotland)
10	Age of criminal responsibility (England and Wales)
13	Minimum age for employment
14	Own an air rifle
	Pay adult fare on public transport
16	Leave school
	Age of sexual consent (heterosexual and homosexual*)
	Buy cigarettes
	Marry (Scotland)
	Marry with parental consent (England and Wales)
	Hold a licence to drive a moped
	Eligible for full employment
17	Hold a licence to drive a car
18	Vote in elections
	Buy alcohol
	Watch films and videos classified as '18'
	Homosexual age of sexual consent
	Marry without parental consent (England and Wales)
25	Adult levels of Income Support
26	Adult in Housing Benefit rules

Source: Pilcher 1995: 62, Table 4.1.
* Homosexual age of consent was reduced to 16 years in 2000 after much public debate. (Sexual Offences (Amendment) Act 2000: 'Age of consent and abuse of a position of trust'.)

The high degree of variability demonstrated in Table 3.1 suggests that there is no agreed point in a child's life when childhood ends and adulthood begins. This is not a politically neutral state of affairs. On the contrary, there has been (and will undoubtedly continue to be) contestation over particular areas within this. Two recent examples of this include the campaign waged throughout 1998 to try to persuade the UK Parliament to standardise the age of sexual consent to sixteen years for both homosexual and heterosexual sexual intercourse; and the dispute over the age of criminal responsibility which re-emerged with the conviction of two ten-year-old boys for the murder of two-year-old James Bulger in 1993. (I will discuss this more fully later in the chapter.)

Regulations concerning the minimum school leaving age and entitlement to welfare benefits serve as indicators about current societal expectations of the boundary between childhood and adulthood. Nevertheless, there are discernible differences even here. The childhood of a middle-class child is expected typically to continue at least to university and often beyond, evidenced by the reduction in grants for students in higher education (Roberts and Sachdev 1996). Similarly, the removal of entitlement to social security benefits for sixteen- to eighteen-year olds has increased the dependency of all children on parents and reduced their scope for self-sufficiency. In contrast, the childhood of a child who has experienced family breakdown and has been 'looked after' by the local authority ends at eighteen years of age in Scotland (twenty-one in England and Wales) when the young person is expected to be old enough to look after her or himself. (See Children (Scotland) Act 1995, Children Act 1989.)

A consideration of official reaction to children involved in prostitution demonstrates society's uncertainty over the boundary between childhood and adulthood, and a major degree of ambivalence towards children and childhood. Children as young as ten years of age have been cautioned for soliciting for the purposes of prostitution, and many more aged fourteen and over have been convicted of similar offences (Home Office figures, England and Wales, quoted in Lee and O'Brien 1995). Yet the behaviour of these children, if witnessed in the context of the family rather than the street, would be liable to be viewed as indicative of sexual abuse rather than prostitution. Childcare agencies have been campaigning to encourage the police to see these children as victims of crime rather than criminals (*Community Care*, 19–25 November 1998: 9).

Kelly *et al.* (1995) point out that there is no consensus on an international level about a definition of childhood. The United Nations

Convention on the Rights of the Child has developed a set of recommendations in response to the sexual exploitation of children, which its signatories are obligated to fulfil. These recommendations are framed under the assumption that childhood is defined as up to eighteen years of age and young people as eighteen to twenty-one years. Yet Kelly *et al.* point out that few countries use these definitions, and as a result it is unlikely that information is kept locally or nationally using these classifications.

Historical accounts of childhood

Historical analyses of childhood (offered by both historians and sociologists) are useful for our consideration for three main reasons. First, they provide further evidence with which to challenge the idea that there is a distinct chronological time which we can point to and call 'childhood'. Second, they make it clear that contemporary ideas of childhood as a time of separateness and difference from adult activities and preoccupations cannot be taken for granted. Third, the disputes that occur between those interested in historical perspectives demonstrate that the study of childhood is, in Frost and Stein's language, an 'ideological battleground'; studies of childhood, like studies of the family, thus reflect a political agenda (1989: 16).

It was the French historian Philippe Aries (1962), who first drew attention to the idea that childhood, rather than being 'natural' or innate, was socially constructed, and that attitudes to childhood changed over time (Gittins 1998: 26). Aries contrasts what he sees as indifference to children (or 'ignorance of childhood') in the tenth century with the 'obsession' with childhood in modern societies. He writes:

> In medieval society the idea of childhood did not exist; this is not to suggest that children were neglected, forsaken or despised. The idea of childhood is not to be confused with affection for children: it corresponds to an awareness of the particular nature of childhood, that particular nature which distinguishes it from the adult, even the young adult. In medieval society, this awareness was lacking. That is why, as soon as the child could live without the constant solicitude of his mother ... he belonged to adult society.
>
> (1962: 125)

Aries based his ideas on the portrayal of children in medieval paintings and poetry. Here children from about five years of age could be found wearing adult clothes and taking part in the full range of adult activities. They were, Aries contends, to all intents and purposes small adults, and, given high rates of child mortality, parents had no special emotional attachment to their children. Aries identifies a shift from the end of the thirteenth century, as children became increasingly differentiated from adults, with their own clothing, literature and activities. The advent of formal education outside the home in the sixteenth and seventeenth centuries then consolidated the concept of childhood as a distinct phenomenon. Aries identifies two distinct dimensions to the new consciousness about childhood: first, he describes a new awareness of, and enjoyment in children by adults; and second, he outlines a new conceptualisation of childhood as a time for physical, intellectual and social development.

Aries is clear that the new understandings about childhood did not impact on all children at the same time. On the contrary, he perceives marked class and gender differences in the experiences of children. It was the new middle classes, he maintains, who were in the forefront of the drive to introduce education for boys. Upper-class boys in the sixteenth and seventeenth centuries received little formal schooling and could be army officers by the age of fourteen and even as young as eleven years on occasions. Aries reports that girls from all classes had no formal schooling and many were married and running households by fourteen years of age. By the eighteenth century, most aristocratic children (both boys and girls) received some schooling, though girls' education finished earlier than boys. Working-class children continued to work to supplement family incomes late into the nineteenth century, and to have life experiences which were very similar to those of their parents. What this suggests is that the construction of childhood as a special category was targeted first and foremost at middle-class boys; subsequently, other children have been accommodated into this characterisation at different times and to different degrees.

Aries locates the lengthening of childhood in changes in ideological beliefs. The Reformation had brought with it ideas about a disciplined life, while Calvinism had stressed the notion of original sin: children were doomed to depravity unless controlled and trained by parents and schools. Then in the eighteenth century, Enlightenment ideas placed on members of society the responsibility that they should seek to contribute to the good of society through attaining rationality: education was to play a major part in this.

Frost and Stein state that Aries' work has been 'central in helping us to build a conception of the historical variability of Western childhood' (1989: 12). There are, however, a number criticisms of Aries' work, criticisms which suggest that he may have been mistaken in his ideas that children joined adult society at the age of five years, or that parents were less attached emotionally to their children in the past (Pollock 1987). Sociologists such as Thane (1981) argue that Aries underplayed both the importance of the Renaissance and its new ideas of individualism, and the significance of economic change and more specifically, the rise of capitalism. Thane links the emergence of modern age groups firmly to the birth and development of European capitalism. She argues that the new middle classes were striving to maximise their control over their wealth and property; adult life too was becoming more demanding, so that more skill was required for those directly involved in commerce or in professional occupations such as the law. The consequence of these two motivating factors was the emergence of schooling and the lengthening of childhood. These pressures were, according to Thane, felt less acutely by both landowners and by the landless labouring poor. Thane suggests that it was only when landowners felt the pressure of competition for power and wealth from the rising middle classes, and later still, when changes in economic and work practices led to the need for a different kind of worker, both literate and numerate, that education became more widely available. By the end of the nineteenth century, the new fear of the 'dangerous classes' led to the introduction of both factory and education legislation aimed at taking working-class children out of the adult world of work and into the children's world of school. Thane concludes that there was a clear correspondence between the birth of capitalism, modern classes and modern age groups (1981: 11).

This account confirms that childhood is not only historically variable, but also varies across gender and class groupings. Jamieson and Toynbee's (1992) sociological investigation of children growing up in rural communities in Scotland between 1900 and 1930 sheds further light on the real-life complexities which are concealed by the catch-all concept 'childhood'. Jamieson and Toynbee contend that a major feature in the lives of children of crofters and farm servants in the early years of the twentieth century was not separateness from adults as we might have anticipated. Instead, children's lives were characterised by continuities between themselves and adults: they rose at the same time, worked together, and went to bed at the same time. Children had few toys and were expected to perform a variety of tasks for their parents, both inside and outside the house. Income earned by children was not for their personal consumption: it was a contribution to the family economy. Household membership carried with it 'expectations of contributing one's labour, in the same way that membership of the community created ties of economic and social reciprocity' (1992: 31). Explaining the implications of this more fully, Jamieson and Toynbee write:

> these children had no childhood in the sense we understand the word today – as a particular special time free from the responsibilities of adulthood, deserving tolerance and indulgence from adults, and allowing time to develop one's potential as an individual. Parents had limited freedom to choose how their children should be brought up; the economic circumstances of some parents demanded that they use what resources they had to survive, in particular the services of their children in the household and whatever else they could be usefully sent to earn. Few parents could afford to give their children treats in the form of pocket money, toys or excursions, even if they wanted to. And very few parents would have been comfortable with the laxity of allowing their children to behave as they wished, not least because this would fly in the face of convention.
>
> (1992: 166)

Although there may have been similarities between the lives of children and adults, however, they were not the same. On closer inspection, it is evident that there was a clear demarcation between what were regarded as 'children's' and 'adults' ' tasks; and within this, differences too between the jobs of boys and girls, reflecting the division of labour between adult men and women. Boys did not drive cattle, look after cows or fetch water, but were expected to tether rogue sheep; girls never did this. Fishing was an exclusively male activity, and it was rare for men or boys to do housework. Jamieson and Toynbee (1992) outline the pattern of work connected with the collection of peat as an example of the age and gender divisions. It was men's job to mark and cut the peat; women's to carry it home; and children's to stack it.

We can now argue that childhood is historically variable, it differs across class and gender, and that there are important continuities in experience between adults and children across generations. In an earlier publication, Jamieson and Toynbee (1990) pinpoint the post-Second World War period as a key moment in the creation of a new idea of childhood and a new relationship between parents and children. Changes in the nature and distribution of goods for consumption in the period after the end of the Second World War meant that working-class 'children's jobs' (daily shopping, collecting fuel, cleaning cutlery, polishing brasses) largely disappeared. At the same time, many more women were working, so that work around the home became a 'main leisure time activity for a significant minority of men and women' (1990: 95). New ideas also emerged in the relationship between adults and children, with parents seeking a more democratic relationship with their children, in contrast to the more authoritarian attitudes of the past. Jamieson and Toynbee locate these changes in increased affluence, the cult of leisure and the development of mass consumption, mass media and mass culture: the shift to the 'affluent consumer society' was associated 'not only with the multiplication of goods provided for children by parents, but also a reduction in the contributions made by children and young people to their family household' (1990: 102).

These historical accounts demonstrate that any idea of childhood as a fixed, chronological period with a universal, agreed conceptualisation is untenable. In practice, childhood as it is currently envisaged in Western society may be a comparatively recent phenomenon, created by shifts in the socio-economic and political world, as well as by psychological ideas about the 'needs' of children as distinct from adults. A historical analysis, however, also demonstrates significant points of connection and overlap between the experiences of adults and children. This leads Frost and Stein (1989) to assert that there is no such thing as a single history of childhood. Instead, there have always been diverse experiences of childhood across class, culture and geography and diverse accounts of family life, illustrating the capacity for both affection and cruelty across generations (1989: 18). Cross-cultural studies extend the discussion further.

Cross-cultural differences in childhood

I have already stated that poverty and wealth have a major impact on children's experiences of childhood throughout the world. In addition, cross-cultural studies suggest that there are widespread differences in child-rearing and in the social organisation of childhood in different cultural and ethnic settings. Some of the key differences are reported by Hill and Tisdall (1997) in their review of anthropological studies. Hill and Tisdall identify that, while in some cultures children spend considerable amounts of time apart from adults, in others children are involved from an early age in work-related activities alongside adults. (This confirms our earlier observations about children in rural Scotland in the early years of the twentieth century.) Research also highlights communities across the world in which the care of young children, rather than being restricted to a nuclear family model, is shared among a wide set of people, often female kinfolk. Hill and Tisdall suggest that ideas of family identity in these settings may be more important than those of individual personality (1997: 16). Hill and Tisdall also point to societies in West Africa where it is common practice to foster children from five years onwards with relatives. This is not perceived to be an act of rejection on behalf of parents (as a white European perspective might assume), but is instead valued as a positive service to the children, who are able to gain wider social links as well as specific skills.

Rogers (1989) considers the varied experiences of children growing up in minority ethnic families in the United Kingdom, and finds that their expectations and norms about what childhood is may at times be very different to the traditional white, Eurocentric model. Although it is important that we should not fall into the trap of stereotyping black families, it is nevertheless also important to draw attention to the continuing reality that there are different ways of thinking about children and childhood. Rogers suggests that traditional families whose origins are in South Asia have ideas about independence and dependence which are deeply at variance with white norms, so that group loyalty and interdependence are valued far more highly than independence and individual freedom (conventionally seen as attributes of being 'grown up'). Children may be expected to contribute in some way towards the management of the household and even the family business at an early age. There may be significant differences in terms of expectations of girls and boys, with girls and boys spending increasingly segregated time as they grow up, girls with their adult female relatives and boys with their adult male relatives. Again this is at odds with expectations about age-specific activities in a conventional white childhood.

Hill and Tisdall (1997) stress the impact of growing up in a racist society on black and minority ethnic children in the UK. They may grow up legally, and in some respects culturally, British but have their own distinctive religious and cultural influences – influences which are routinely marginalised, discounted and discriminated against (1997: 17). This means that for them, oppression and discrimination may be a large part of their experience of childhood. Meera Syal (1996), in a deeply evocative novel, tells the story of a black girl from a Punjabi family growing up in a white mining community in the English Midlands in the 1960s. The girl at the centre of the story moves in and out of different social and cultural groups at home, at school and in the neighbourhood, as she successfully negotiates her passage from childhood into adulthood.

Summary

I have argued that the idea of childhood as a specific age grouping is not sustainable. An investigation of differences between children socially, culturally and historically reveals that childhood is a socially and historically specific construction; definitions vary between classes, ethnic groupings and genders as well as across time. James and Prout (1990) put this succinctly:

> Childhood is understood as a social construction ... Childhood, as distinct from biological immaturity, is neither a natural nor universal feature of human groups but appears as a specific structural and cultural component of many societies. Childhood is a variable of social analysis. It can never be entirely divorced from other variables such as class, gender or ethnicity. Comparative and cross-cultural analysis reveals a variety of childhoods rather than a single and universal phenomenon.
>
> (1990: 8)

Implications for practice

The summary suggests that, as social workers, we should examine where *our* ideas about childhood are coming from, so that we can give proper attention to the differing childhoods of the children with whom we are working. This is not to recommend a cultural relativism which seeks to play down potentially damaging or abusive experiences. Rather it is about an acknowledgement that the happy, free, play-focused childhood of television advertisements is a particular kind of myth: it is a story that we tell ourselves which has little basis in the reality of children's lives. As social workers, we are expected to make assessments and recommendations on behalf of children. We must do so from an understanding of both the diversity of children's experiences and the ways in which children's lives are structured by age, gender, class and ethnicity.

But there is another, sobering point to be made here; one which suggests that we should consider childhood in a more global sense. Harris (1989) reminds us that much of the comfort

and material wealth of the developed world is based on the
reality of child labour and poverty wages in developing countries.
Harris writes:

> if child protection were indeed based on considerations
> other than law and policy – on a hierarchy of need or
> suffering, for example – it is inconceivable that we should be
> so exercised by the murder of a single Maria Colwell or
> Jasmine Beckford yet be so acquiescent in the systematic
> destruction of young lives in more distant parts of the globe.
>
> (1989 : 29)

Sociology and childhood: traditional perspectives

Hockey and James (1993) point out that when we think about
childhood, we tend to see it not as a entity in its own right, but
instead as a preparation for adulthood, that is, for what is regarded
as *the* central stage of the life course. Socialisation into adulthood
therefore becomes a key sociological concern. Socialisation is
commonly presented as 'the process whereby individuals in a society
absorb the values, standards and beliefs current in that society'
(Coleman 1992: 13). Two major perspectives have dominated socialisation theory: the normative perspective, which locates power within
societal structures, and the interpretive paradigm, which locates
power within the individual. Grbich (1990) identifies a third position developing, one which comprises various conceptualisations of
the two, viewing both individual and society as potentially powerful
(1990: 517).

The normative perspective

For those working from a normative paradigm, socialisation is viewed
as a passive process over which we have little or no control. For functionalists such as Durkheim and Parsons, it is seen to be achieved by
the internalisation of commonly-held, societal values and norms
through the agency of the family, school, community, workplace, etc.
A Marxist or radical feminist viewpoint assumes that it is enforced on
individuals by the regulatory mechanisms of society, such as the courts,

police, education system, etc., which reward certain behaviours and punish others or through the workings of patriarchy and the sexual division of labour. Socialisation is thus envisaged as a mechanism either for transmitting the social consensus or for enforcing social conformity. It is concerned with the social and cultural forces which impinge on us from birth, beginning with 'primary socialisation' in the family (as the child learns how to behave through the intimate relationships of the family) and progressing to 'secondary socialisation' which occurs in the school, peer group and wider community, as the child (and later adult) learns to deal with and become a member of the outside world.

This conceptualisation of the socialisation process has been criticised for being determinist and absolutist in emphasis. For example, in an influential essay, Wrong (1961) describes this as an 'over-socialized conception of man'. Critics have pointed out that socialisation is never a one-way street; there are always counter-cultures at odds with the 'dominant' view. Willis' celebrated study of working-class boys (1977) takes issue with those who see school as an inculcator of middle-class values that are supposedly absorbed unconsciously by working-class children. He points instead to the vast numbers of kids who do not conform, and who actively resist attempts to incorporate them into a dominant middle-class culture. He argues that for many children, their counter-culture is what matters most, and that this is a working-class culture with profound similarities to shop-floor culture. This is not a defeated culture, but one which has rules and skills all of its own.

The interpretive perspective

The normative perspective, I have suggested, minimises individual 'agency' and the capacity of the individual to interact with and influence his or her social environment. Interpretive sociologists, in contrast, present socialisation as an interactive process. It is still accepted that we enter a pre-given social world, but individuals are no longer seen as wholly constrained by societal structures. Instead, it is pointed out that individuals (children and adults) try out new behaviour and build on previous experiences of given situations, bringing meaning and purpose to their actions.

American social psychologist George Herbert Mead (1934) has had a major influence on thinking about the interactive nature of the socialisation process. He argues that there is no 'self' or personality that exists at birth. Instead, the self is constituted throughout life, confirmed and transformed by a sequence of negotiations with others who are themselves on life's journey. The 'self' has two components: first, the self is subject ('I') as we initiate social reaction; and second, the self is object ('me'), because in taking the role of another, we form impressions of ourselves. Social experience is thus the interplay of the 'I' and the 'me: our actions are spontaneous yet guided by how others respond to us (Macionis and Plummer 1997: 138). Socialisation is understood as the process of learning to take the role of the other; Mead suggests that this process continues throughout life, as changing social circumstances reshape who we are.

Symbolic interactionists leading on from Mead stress the importance of the 'roles' which we play: the primary task for a child in order to make sense of, and influence, the world is to learn to take the role of the 'other' (for example, mother, father, sibling). By adapting and submitting to the demands of the social world, the child learns to become a role player in different settings at different times. It is argued that each of us learns a slightly different combination of roles that will always be defined in slightly different ways (see Berger and Luckmann 1967).

Some sociologists, however, have criticised what is seen as over-determinism in the presentation of roles and how they work. Connell (1983), for example, argues that, because we all hold countless roles, all of which have different expectations of them, no generalisations can be made here. He also disputes the claim that role (and the idea of internalisation of role prescriptions) can explain social learning and personality formation. He writes that role cannot explain 'the opposition with which social pressure is met – the girls who become tomboys, the women who become lesbians, the shoppers who become shoplifters, the citizens who become revolutionaries' (1983: 202). In other words, role cannot explain resistance. Goffman is also interested in the ways that people actively resist, refuse or manipulate their given roles. In his (1968) study of asylums he argues that even in institutions with the most rigid rules, there is still a process of negotiation: a twisting of the rules, an unwritten contract between warder and patient.

Socialisation as a map

This leads us to Grbich's third conceptualisation of socialisation: that it is a map, not a blueprint; it can never be a single, total process, and expectations others have of us will always be conflicting, loose and obscure, differing from situation to situation. There are also many areas of life where there are no established rules and expectations, where we have to make independent assessments. In the 'postmodern' world, socialisation can never be a complete, all-encompassing process. Bauman (1990) writes:

> Being free and unfree at the same time is perhaps the most common of our experiences. It is also, arguably, the most confusing ... much in the history of sociology may be explained as an on-going effort to solve this puzzle.
>
> (1990: 20)

Bauman goes on to explore more fully the idea of freedom and independence. We are free to make choices and decisions, but the choices and decisions which we can make are constrained in various ways: by those who set the rules about the choices we can make; by qualifications and personal resources, financial and otherwise; by class, gender, ethnicity. The groups of which we are members enable us to be free and at the same time constrain us by drawing borders on that freedom. It is therefore important to ask whose interests are being met in the sustaining of particular class, gender and racial inequalities. There needs to be an adequate analysis of how power works in society; of how the status quo is maintained and why.

The fundamental question for sociologists now changes. Instead of asking 'how does society socialise individuals?' it is necessary to ask 'who socialises society?' This raises much larger questions about the ways in which society works: about whose interests are met in the status quo, with all its particular class, gender and racial inequalities. Writing about gender socialisation, Mackie (1987) argues that gender, age, and sexuality are all social constructs that are built upon relatively minor biological and psychological differences between the sexes. The main purpose of gender socialisation, in her view, is to perpetuate the inequality between women and men. A host of agencies are involved in this process: the mass media, films, newspapers, employers, governments, the law, the education system, the police, social workers. (See also Sharpe 1976 and Lees 1986 on the ways that girls learn to be women.)

While I wholly accept that gender inequalities are structured into society, I find this approach too pessimistic, ignoring as it does the potential for contradictory discourse and the importance of resistance. Historical studies of socialisation and the creation of gender identity demonstrate that what is considered permissible behaviour for women and men has changed considerably in the last fifty years or so (Moore

1993). It has changed too at particular moments because of political exigencies such as the Second World War, where women found themselves in many positions in society formerly occupied only by men. Women today receive very mixed messages about their rightful situation. They are encouraged onto the labour market to carry out what are often low-paid, part-time insecure jobs. At the same time, government cutbacks have led to a reduction in nursery places, and community care planning has been built on an assumption that women will continue to be primary carers (Finch 1984). (This issue is discussed more fully in Chapter 6.)

A parallel point can be made about cultural specificity in relation to gender socialisation. Different cultures have assumed different role models for women and men. Men have not always been hunters and gatherers, just as women have not always been principally involved in childcare. There has been extensive anthropological research in this area (e.g. Oakley 1972). Studies of masculinity have similarly indicated that there are many different ways of behaving 'like a man' across cultures. Tolson (1977) demonstrates that definitions of 'masculine' conduct vary between cultures and societies, hence Italian men are allowed (and encouraged) to be emotional and passionate while English men are expected to be inexpressive and cold.

Brittan and Maynard (1984) are also interested in the origins of socialisation, in this case, the ways in which children acquire racist and sexist beliefs and attitudes. Brittan and Maynard argue that racism and sexism exist not because of socialisation; on the contrary, 'socialisation reproduces what is already there' (1984: 111). This does not lead them, however, to be despairing about change. Instead, they point to the capacity of Black Power and Black Consciousness movements in the United States and South Africa to reclaim negative images of what it is to be black in a racist society and recreate them in a powerful and positive way.

Summary

I have argued that there are pitfalls in a sociological perspective which is only interested in children as 'becoming adults'. This approach may undermine the importance of conceptualising childhood as a social category, and may lead us to undervalue children as social actors in their own right. In addition, normative sociological theories of socialisation are inherently conservative: as Mayall states, they assume that society is a 'given', and that children are 'to be taught how to fit in' (1996: 54). I have stressed that socialisation is better understood as a two-way process: we (as children and as adults) interact with the world as it does with us. Socialisation should not be seen as a stereotyping, for we are all different, and bring to every situation our unique age, gender, ethnic, cultural, class, familial and historical position. This means that we should not make assumptions based on our own experiences of socialisation. Instead, we should be open to the possibilities which individual history and agency, structural position and cultural differences bring. Moreover, an analysis of power is essential in understanding the paradox of freedom and dependence.

Implications for practice

As agencies of socialisation, social work and probation organisations should be clear about the potential they have for either perpetuating inequalities or encouraging new attitudes and behaviours. We know from studies of decision-making in social work that there are widespread differences in the assessment of, and interventions with, girls and boys (Campbell 1981, Hudson 1988), just as black children's experiences of the childcare system have been very different to those of white children (Ahmed 1989, Barn 1993). It is our responsibility to do something about this.

Denzin (1987) describes the contemporary postmodern child as 'a media child': 'he or she is cared for by the television set, in conjunction with the day-care center. Cultural myths are learned from television, including how to be violent and how to be a man in violent society' (1987: 33). Social workers – themselves part of society – have an important job to do in trying to support what they perceive to be more positive images and identities for children and young people.

Sociology and childhood: more recent perspectives

Since the mid 1980s, there has been an explosion of interest in the sociology of childhood as sociologists have sought to redefine children as the subjects of research and at the same time understand the ways in which childhood is socially constructed by adult society. There is still much work to be done here: Chisholm suggests that the sociology of childhood is still very much 'in its own infancy' (Chisholm *et al.* 1990: 5). Nevertheless, a number of key debates of relevance to social work and childcare emerge in the new sociological interest in childhood and children. These include:

- The regulation of childhood.
- Childhood – lengthening or disappearing?
- Children – individual consumers or members of an oppressed class?
- Children – angels or demons?

The regulation of childhood

Ennew (1986) argues that the most important feature of childhood today is the idea of 'separateness'. She sees this in two parts: first, the idea that children should be 'quarantined' away from various 'nasty infections' of adulthood, such as sex, violence and commerce; and second, the notion that childhood should be a happy, innocent, free stage of life – a time of play and socialisation, rather than work and economic responsibility (1986: 33).

The notion of childhood as something separate from adulthood is, as we have already considered, a relatively new phenomenon. Children in the UK in the middle of the nineteenth century lived lives that were much closer to those of their parents, working, eating and sleeping together, with little scope for play or age-segregated recreation. With industrialisation and urbanisation came the creation of a new wage-earning class, and with this, a concern about the behaviour and habits of what became known as the 'dangerous' classes (Pearson 1983). Children, themselves a constituent part of the new working class, were central to this concern. Factory legislation to limit the working hours of children and women was accompanied by legislation to introduce full-time education for all children. Children were literally swept off the streets and into new controlled settings: schools, reformatories, children's homes and youth organisations. The impulse to prevent the contamination of urban poverty and delinquency was so strong that thousands of city children were 'rescued' from their old worlds and either 'boarded out' with families in remote crofts and farms (see Abrams 1998) or transported to the 'new' worlds of Canada, Australia, New Zealand and South Africa.[3]

Pearson (1983) argues that it is not simply the behaviour of children that changes over time, but public reaction to that behaviour. In his vivid account of the nineteenth-century moral panics about working-class children, he demonstrates that what had previously been regarded as 'normal' childhood activity became criminalised. For example, it had in the past been considered acceptable, 'normal' behaviour for children to sell goods in the street. But during the nineteenth century, this behaviour became relabelled as delinquent and punishable.[4] From this he infers that an examination of 'bad' children tells us more about current perceptions of safety, 'dangerousness' and law and order than it does about children and young people themselves.

Although Foucault was not primarily interested in a study of childhood as such, his analysis of what he sees as a shift in disciplinary mechanisms in society (1977) provides further information about the development of childhood as a distinct, regulated phase. Foucault identifies a shift in techniques of punishment from the surveillance of bodies to the surveillance of minds; from the control of the problem to the control of the problem-doer (the individual or the family); from a traditional form of law based on juridical rights to a colonisation by the 'psy' complex (psychological and psychiatric ideas and practices) and the criteria of 'normalisation'. The 'psy' discourse, according to Foucault, created the categories which it then used to classify and divide up individuals, and regulate and control behaviour.

Donzelot (1980), working from Foucault's ideas, examines the development in the late eighteenth and early nineteenth centuries of a sector which he defines as 'the social'; neither public nor private, independent from and connected with other sectors (juridical, educational, economic and political). A new series of professions assembled under the common banner of 'social work' and took over the mission of 'civilising the social body' (1980: 96). As a consequence, children and the family are 'policed' today to a degree that would have been unimaginable one hundred years ago. Teachers, health visitors, social workers, youth leaders, counsellors, psychiatrists, ministers of religion, childcare 'experts' all have a say in regulating childhood and in maintaining children as innocent, asexual, dependent and in need of protection, as do education and welfare systems. Theories of child development and socialisation thus constitute the childhood which we take for granted at the same time as they set the parameters for 'normal' and 'abnormal' children's behaviour: in Foucault's conceptualisation, they create childhood.

It is not only ideas about childcare that have set the boundaries of childhood. Parton (1985) argues that child abuse tragedies have played a major part in educating society about what childhood is and should be. Over the last twenty-five years since the public enquiry in 1973 into the death of Maria Colwell, there have been almost forty public enquiries in the UK into child abuse. These enquiries have presented good parenting and the love of children as the norm; any deviations from this have been presented as individual aberrations which should be treated as such. The focus for social workers working with families and children has therefore been to identify the small numbers of children who are seen as 'at risk' in families, and allocate resources accordingly (see also Rodger 1996).

Reviewing this period, Parton *et al.* (1997) suggest that a shift has taken place from child abuse being constituted as an essentially medico-social reality with the expertise of doctors as central, to a new position where it is now seen as a socio-legal problem, with legal expertise as pre-eminent (1997: 19). At the same time, there has been a move away from a discourse centred on child *abuse* to one which is built around the much broader idea of child *protection*: not only the protection of the child, but also 'the protection of parents and family privacy from unwarranted state interventions' (1997: 41).

This can be understood as the latest compromise position in a battle which has been fought over the last hundred and fifty years or so between those who have wished to promote greater state involvement in the lives of families and children and those who have believed that regulation was a matter for the individual, not the state (Cree 1995).[5]

Childhood – lengthening or disappearing?

While childhood has been constituted as a separate phase, so children's dependent state has been stretched far longer than in the past: although children may reach puberty at ten or eleven years, they may not be seen to enter adulthood until finishing full-time education aged twenty-one and upwards. Sociological studies in recent years have sought to explore this so-called lengthening of childhood: to examine children's activities in school, employment and leisure, their relationships with older generations, their dependency and independence, their legal status, and the impact of gender, 'race' and class (see Chisholm *et al.* 1990, Coleman 1992, Mayall 1994, Qvortrup *et al.* 1994). This research demonstrates that children's lives have become increasingly age-segregated and partitioned off from those of adults, thus increasing both their isolation and their dependency. Moreover, children are spending more and more time in institutional and organised settings, from pre-school to school and after-school care. As a consequence, they can be understood as inhabiting a separate and exclusive sphere in which they are protected from, and at the same time controlled by, the adult world.

Ennew (1994) sees connections between the 'curricularization' of children's lives and the compartmentalised lives inhabited by adults.

Just as adults move from different spheres of home, work, shopping and leisure, so the school timetable has been extended outside the walls of the classroom and into the whole of children's existence. Ennew identifies this as a feature of modern lives: 'Leisure and play, far from being separate and different from work, are now timetabled according to the same criteria and the same units of time' (1994:132). The curricularising of children's lives increases both the protection of children and their dependence on adults, as adults ferry children to and from the various cultural and sporting activities which fill their out-of-school hours. Within their tight schedules, Ennew argues, children make superficial and fragmented social relationships with other children and adults, and the idea of 'free time' disappears as children are confronted with the imperative to organise and structure their time 'constructively'. Qvortrup (1995) suggests that, from this perspective, childhood is becoming a shorter and shorter phase of a person's life (1995: 195).

Ennew's account has clear resonance for the lives of many middle-class children living in western Europe or the United States. How transferable the scenario is to working-class children and parents in the same countries is less certain. Families on low incomes and without transport will be much less able to make use of the many and varied social and cultural activities which are routinely available to more mobile, middle-class families with much greater disposable income. Because of this, working-class children are much more likely to continue to take part in unsupervised play around their streets and neighbourhoods. In addition, there is some research evidence that it is middle-class families who make most use of external childcare resources such as nurseries and paid child-minders. Working-class families still rely more heavily for childcare on the extended family network, including parents, siblings and close neighbours, suggesting that the influence of family members (rather than paid adult carers) may continue to be prominent in their lives (Hill 1987).

Studies of children's unsupervised play activities demonstrate the continuing vibrancy of the parts of children's lives that have not yet been colonised by adults. Opie's research (1993) into children at play suggests that games, rhymes, jokes and songs in streets and playgrounds are still an important part of childhood. In addition, Ennew (1994) identifies a small number of studies which suggest that children will resist and take charge of their own time, in whatever ways they can. The main force of their resistance, she argues, is to hide from adults what they do in their own time: that is, what children do when they tell us they are doing 'nothing'.

Children involved in unstructured play continue, however, to be seen as a threat to others and to themselves. The curfew on children under ten years of age playing outside after 9 p.m. first introduced in 1997 to three council housing estates in the town of Hamilton, in Scotland, and extended in 1998 to other cities in the UK bears witness both to a continuing street life for working-class children, as well as to public anxiety about the potential 'dangerousness' for children of unrestricted time, particularly unscheduled time in the evenings (*Community Care*, 5–11 November 1998). [6]

Boyden (1990) is highly critical of the ways in which the 'official' Western view of childhood is being disseminated internationally to countries and cultures which may traditionally have very different ideas about the capabilities and competencies of children. Children on the streets, out of school and away from home are being targeted for intervention by welfare and aid agencies. Yet the activities of these children may be understood as mechanisms of survival, performing the important function of preparing them for adult life.

Postman (1983) has very different ideas about childhood in modern industrial societies. Far from lengthening, he argues, childhood is in fact disappearing, because the dividing line between childhood and adulthood is being rapidly eroded. Postman sees this as a wholly disagreeable state of affairs. He illustrates his argument by pointing to the children who commit 'adult' crimes and the increasing similarities between the worlds of children and adults: schools are becoming indistinguishable from places of work, and adults and children now share the same consumer culture. Postman blames the media, and in particular television, for this state of affairs, because television has removed the 'mysteries and secrets' which kept children innocent and separate from the adult world. Historical analysis suggests that Postman is wrong: that some children have in the past committed 'adult' crimes (Pearson 1983) and that children have not always been kept apart from adult sexuality (Aries 1962). Nevertheless, there does seem to be widespread agreement amongst sociologists that there has been a 'blurring of the category of childhood', visible not only in children's activities, but also in the current debates about the interests and rights of children, and in arguments which press for the independence, the enfranchisement and the economic autonomy of children (Jenks 1996: 119). This perspective will be explored more fully in the next section.

Children – individual consumers or members of an exploited class?

As childhood has become more regulated, and as children's lives have been seen to adopt patterns which resemble more closely those of adults, so some sociologists have stressed the increasing individualisation of childhood; others have explored the emergence of children as a separate, exploited class.

Frones (1994) argues that childhood has become more individualised: as children's lives have become increasingly compartmentalised, they have become consumers in their own right, with their own special clothes, books, games and television programmes. Frones locates this development in the context of the emergence of the individual in modern society. This process, he suggests, involves two dimensions: individuation (that is, the tendency of the modern state and organisational system to treat the individual as the basic unit) and individualisation (that is, an emphasis on the individual as a psychological personality) (1994: 147).

Frones argues that the individualisation of children is a postwar development, which can be identified first with teenagers and then later with ever-younger groups of children. Qvortrup (1995) puts this graphically:

> children are being individualised in a way themselves – exactly as parents and other adults have been individualised. Children spend more and more time as representatives for themselves rather than for their family; they have their own ID-card, their own key, their own money, and some experiments have already been made with plastic cards to be used each day for children in kindergartens to control children's time use for economic reasons.
>
> (1995: 196)

The individualisation process can be clearly demonstrated in the movement for children's rights. From the 1970s onwards, campaigners for child liberation have fought for children to be treated the same as other people (that is, adults), with the same rights and privileges, including the right to vote, work, own property, and rights to make sexual and guardianship choices. In contrast, others have argued that children cannot be seen as self-determining agents; they cannot make rational choices and adults must therefore make decisions in their best interests (Archard, 1993, calls this the 'caretaker thesis').

Pilcher (1995: 50) claims that the 'liberationist' perspective is gaining ground. She evidences this in the emergence of organisations which seek to listen to children's grievances, such as Childline; in the redefinition of corporal punishment as physical violence; and in the legislation which promotes the rights of the child (for example, the Children Act of 1989, the United Nations Convention on the Rights of the Child by which the UK government in 1991 agreed to be bound).

Oldman (1994) presents a very different approach. He argues that children's experience is best understood as the experience of a subordinate class, exploited by an adult class. Their activities are structured so as to serve the economic interests of adults; their work at home and school is no less 'work' than that of adults. Oldman suggests that the two basic mechanisms of the exploitation of children by adults are the unsupervised activity of children (which frees parents from childcare) and formal supervision outside the family (which provides adults with paid 'child work'). Ennew (1994) gives support to this conceptualisation. She writes:

> By trivializing childhood activities, marginalizing and economically devalorizing children, adults in industrial societies reproduce the power relations that enable them to take hold of children's time, organize it, curricularize it and simultaneously control the next generation on behalf of an economic system that depends for its very existence on the subdivision of human energy into units of labour time.
>
> (1994: 143)

Social work and children's rights

Although recent childcare legislation in the UK illustrates an acceptance of the idea of children as individuals with rights and choices, how far this has actually developed in practice remains open to question. The Children Act of 1989 and the Children (Scotland) Act of 1995 both place the child at the centre of the legislation. The child's welfare is said to be paramount and must be considered in context of his/her physical, emotional and educational needs, age, gender, background, and the capacity of his/her caregivers to perform their task adequately. There is an imperative on the part of social workers to find out what the child's wishes are – the child's voice must be heard. But there is also an expectation that parents and other significant adults will be given increased respect and consideration, thus giving additional support to the status quo in terms of balance of power between adults and children (Colton *et al.* 1995, Hill and Aldgate 1996, Tisdall 1996). This demonstrates the importance of the context within which childhood takes place. While the rhetoric of childhood may conceptualise the child as a unique person with rights to claim and choices to make, those rights and choices may be executed within the context of a rather circumscribed and limited range of options.

Hill and Tisdall (1997) argue that there are numerous gaps in meeting children's rights in the UK. Far from moving forwards in relation to children's rights for protection and provision, they state that the UK may be seen to be moving backwards, as children's poverty is increasing; more children are unemployed or underemployed; more children are to be found homeless and on the street (1997: 256). Scraton, a Marxist sociologist, is even more critical of the UK's record on human rights for children. He writes:

> whatever the relative material benefits, quality of life and opportunities self-evident within advanced capitalist societies, structural inequalities, ritualized abuse and the systematic denial of citizen's rights to all under the age of 18 are deeply etched into Britain's social and political landscape.
>
> (1997: 179)

Scraton concludes that an analysis of power is the only way forward: adults must address their position as oppressors, and expose 'the dominant lie that adult power and its manifestations are conceived and administered for the benefit of children' (1997: 186).

Children – angels or demons?

Society's ambivalence towards children and childhood is clearly apparent in the categorisation of children as either innocent victims in need of protection ('angels') or bad children from whom society needs protection ('demons'). This dichotomy between children as innocent victims and children as demons or criminals lies at the heart of childcare legislation and practice.

We have already considered Ennew's characterisation of childhood as a time of innocence and separateness from the adult world of sex, violence and work. Those children who do not conform to this stereotype – children who are themselves troublesome and who commit crime – are demonised as delinquent and 'unnatural'. Davis and Bourhill (1997) argue that media portrayal of children's involvement in crime, whether as perpetrators or victims, is 'central in creating and reinforcing public perceptions of childhood. While this has consequences for children, individually and collectively, its derivation lies within a broader context of media and political concern over a perceived breakdown in law and order' (1997: 29). Davis and Bourhill locate attitudes to children who commit crime in the context of the sociological study of moral panics and delinquency, which began with the groundbreaking investigation by Cohen in the early 1970s into the explosion of press attention about Mods and Rockers (Cohen 1972). (This subject is explored more fully in Chapter 4.)

Bringing the discussion up-to-date, Davis and Bourhill assert that the abduction and subsequent murder of two-year-old James Bulger in Liverpool in 1993 by two ten-year-old boys was a key moment which overshadowed all that had gone before. The fact that the killers were children themselves led to a new conceptualisation. Not only were the child killers 'evil', they were indicative of a 'crisis' in childhood. The solutions proposed were, predictably, reactionary and authoritarian, leading to sentences of a minimum of fifteen years' imprisonment for the two boys, and an expansion in secure accommodation for young offenders more generally.

While accepting the general thesis that children who kill become symbols of a breakdown in beliefs about children, human nature and society, the reaction to James Bulger's death was not in fact a wholly new scenario. An earlier incident of child-killing caught the public (and the media) imagination in the same way as the Bulger case. The murder of two boys aged three and four years by Mary Bell in Newcastle in 1968 received as widespread media coverage (though, of course, there were undoubtedly fewer televisions in people's homes at that time). The Mary Bell case continues to exercise public concern, as evidenced in 1998 by the furore over the publication of Bell's biography, *Cries Unheard*, written by Gitta Sereny.[7]

Taking a very different perspective, Gittins (1998) argues that by defining children as 'angels', we create a need for devils, 'because those aspects of children and of ourselves that we cannot accept as good must be directed, projected somewhere else' (1998: xvi). In her analysis of fictional literature, she points to the complex juxtaposition of innocence and guilt, good and evil, light and dark, Christ and the devil. By placing the blame out there, external to ourselves, as 'Other', we hide from the 'cruelty and corruption within ourselves'. She argues that only by facing up to this can we begin to move on and change. Gittins also explores the ways in which children learn and begin to understand about sexuality and adult morality. She suggests that children perceive and understand in different ways from adults, and that by trying to 'protect' children, we may in reality be prolonging not their 'inno-cence', but their 'dependency, ignorance and disempowerment' (1998: 172).

There is one final point to be made in an analysis of children and the idea of innocence. Kitzinger's research (1990) into children who have been sexually abused challenges the mythology around children as innocent, passive victims. She argues that ideas of innocence titillate abusers, stigmatise the knowing child and present an ideology of childhood which is used to deny children power. She demonstrates that children are anything but 'passive victims': they fight back in whatever way they can. This connects with earlier accounts of the importance of an approach to understanding childhood that takes on board issues of both power and resistance.

Implications for practice

I have argued that the way we construct childhood has real consequences, not only for children themselves, but also for the agencies and institutions that work with children. Children are constructed as separate from adults: innocent, vulnerable and unequal. They are also increasingly constructed as individual consumers, with individual preferences and rights, which must be addressed. These developments may be seen to have posi-tive aspects for children who are the subjects of social work intervention. Children who are 'looked after' are now routinely invited to attend care reviews; children's views are sought in both Children's Hearings in Scotland and in divorce courts. But there is a sense in which a sociological imagination urges us not to be complacent about any progress, which may have been made here. Children's rights continue to be exercised in a very limited, controlled setting; any decision-making on the part of children takes place in a firmly adult-led, paternalist environment.

It is also important that we place in context the shift from punitive, corporal punishment in schools and at home to a more disciplinary form of control. Foucault (1977) and Donzelot (1980) have convincingly demonstrated that the removal of punitive measures of control does not necessarily imply a freer society. On the contrary, children's lives in Western societies today, as we have seen, are more tightly regulated and monitored by a whole range of educational and health professionals than ever before. As social workers we play a part in that regulation, whether through voluntary measures of support or through compulsory measures, such as supervision or even the removal of children from home. This is one of the main paradoxes within the social work discourse. Social work is not in practice about care *or* control: it is instead about care *and* control.

There is another point here, however. With its traditional emphasis on individual (and family) pathology, social work with children has paid insufficient attention to issues of culture, class and gender, to discrimination and oppression on the grounds of 'race', sexuality and gender, and to growing inequalities in income and wealth.[8] Children who use social work services are predominantly poor, working-class children, often from lone parent families and from minority ethnic communities. They are also structurally disadvantaged in society on the basis of their age, a reality that social work with children has largely ignored to date.

Conclusion

This chapter has covered a wide range of material in relation to childhood and children. I have argued that childhood is a social and historical construction: that it changes over time, and that it is specific in terms of class, 'race', gender and culture. Traditional sociological theories based on ideas of socialisation and children as 'becoming adults' have been criticised as functionalist and inherently conservative, working from the basis of a white, Western notion of an idealised childhood. I have suggested that more recent sociological perspectives offer new understandings of childhood as a separate, familialised and individualised institution. Because definitions of children and childhood vary historically, socially and culturally, it can be difficult to quantify the nature and extent of the issues faced by children and young people across countries and over time. However, there is an even greater sense that 'our historical perspectives on childhood reflect the changes in the organisation of our social structure' (Jenks 1996: 80). In other words, we build the frameworks that create the very concept of childhood itself.

I have asserted that social work practice with children has in the past betrayed its psychologically based, paternalist and adultist origins. Pringle (1996, 1998) argues even more forcibly that welfare systems may actually reinforce and maintain social oppression rather than challenging it. This is because welfare systems are structured by the same oppressive power dynamics as societies themselves. In his analysis of child welfare systems across Europe, Pringle concludes that both the European model of family support and the English model of child protection fail to address adequately the issues of structural social oppression that characterise the lives of children.

I believe that the ways forward for social work with children lie in a genuine attempt on our part to confront both the diversities of experiences of children, and their shared experience as members of an oppressed group in society. We must then attempt to redress some of the inequalities experienced by children: to seek to empower children to make realistic and positive choices, and at the same time to trust that children, given the freedom and space to be themselves, will spend their time in no less creative ways than we might expect of other human beings. We must also, I believe, seek to challenge poverty and discrimination in the lives of children with whom we are working.[9] By operating from a critically aware, anti-oppressive framework, I believe that there are possibilities for the future in terms of the development of a more empowering practice with children. Waterhouse and McGhee express this well:

> Perhaps the question for the future is not just how we can find those children who are likely to be seriously injured or abused by their carers but how all children in need can be supported and protected in our society.
>
> (1996: 129)

Recommended reading

- Cannan, C. and Warren, C. (1997) *Social Action with Children and Families: A Community Development Approach to Child and Family Welfare*, London: Routledge (a good practice guide for social work with children and families).
- Gittins, D. (1998) *The Child in Question*, Basingstoke: Macmillan (a thought-provoking, personal and well-theorised account).
- Hill, M. and Tisdall, K. (1997) *Children and Society*, Harlow, Essex: Addison Wesley Longman (a useful overview of the subject).

- Mayall, B. (1994) *Children's Childhoods: Observed and Experienced*, London: Falmer Press (an insight into current sociological concerns).
- Scraton, P. (1997) *'Childhood' in 'Crisis'?*, London: UCL Press (an edited collection, with a strong line of argument expressed throughout).

4 Youth

Introduction

In Chapter 3, I argued that the study of childhood and children has been, until recent years, neglected in sociological research and literature. Nothing could be further from the truth when considering sociological interest in youth and young people. There has been a huge investment of sociological time and energy in scrutinising youth, much of this based on the assumption that youth and young people are problems requiring analysis. This chapter aims to 'unpack' ideas of youth as a social problem and young people as 'troubled' and 'troublesome', developing further the thesis that age is best understood not simply as a biological fact, but as a social, historical and cultural construction, mediated by relations of power in society.

The chapter will outline dominant approaches to youth and young people, drawing on influential psychological and sociological approaches that have set the parameters for past and current conceptualisations of youth. It will be argued that our common-sense ideas about youth are created by the coming-together of psychological and sociological discourses which name and set boundaries on expectations and behaviours. The chapter goes on to discuss current themes in the sociology of youth. The chapter begins, as ever, with a question: what is youth?

Definitions of youth

If it is difficult to make absolute claims about childhood as a fixed period in the life-span, then this is even more evident with the notion of youth. For young people in today's Western world, we might expect youth to begin with the start of puberty. But when does puberty start? We know that puberty has lowered by several years because of improvements in diet and living conditions (Osgerby 1998). We also know that puberty is not a single moment and may take years, and how it is interpreted will depend on the society in which it takes place. As Judith Ennew (1986) has identified, the onset of menstruation may be a cause for celebration; it may be ignored completely; or it may be mourned, depending on historical, social and cultural ways of viewing this. Marking the ending of the stage of youth is equally problematic. The young person who leaves home to get married or have a child at sixteen years of age may cease to see him or herself as a youth. At the same time, the student in his or her twenties who is still financially dependent on a parent may experience the feelings of powerlessness and dependency associated with youth for a much longer period of time (Coleman 1992).

Although it may be difficult to pin down youth as a chronological stage, it is without doubt a time in which real changes take place in young people: changes in physical capacities, linguistic and reasoning abilities and in sexual development. Yet no less significant is the context in which these changes are taking place, that is, the political and economic, social and cultural environment which impacts on young people undergoing the transition from childhood dependency to adult independence.

Historical accounts of youth

The period between childhood and adulthood varies considerably across cultures and historical times, as detailed historical work demonstrates. Aries' (1962) inquiry into childhood, as discussed in Chapter 3, suggested that the medieval child in Europe passed from infanthood to adulthood without any intervening phase. In other words, they became adults at the age of five years. Another influential historian, Gillis (1981), looks at this very differently. He does not dispute that it was common practice in pre-industrial Europe for children to leave home at a young age to live in others' households as servants or apprentices. But Gillis argues that this does not imply that they had achieved adulthood. On the contrary, he sees this as evidence of a very long transition period, beginning when the child first became somewhat independent of its family at about eight years of age, to the point of compete independence at marriage or inheritance, ordinarily in the mid to late twenties (1981: 2). Gillis argues therefore that pre-industrial society did recognise a stage in life that was different both from young childhood and adulthood, and he sees this stage as characterised by a long phase of gradually increasing independence from parental control.

Gillis goes on to assert that there were few distinctions between younger and older youth in this extended period of semi-independence, because there was no universal schooling to postpone entry into the world of work, and no clear break at the onset of physical and sexual maturity. Puberty and the menarche came comparatively late in pre-industrial societies (just over seventeen years of age in Norway in 1850), and physical growth was, Gillis maintains, slow, with young people not attaining full physical powers until their mid-twenties. Importantly, Gillis claims that there is no evidence to suggest that there was any difficult or emotionally disruptive time in the teenage years, such that we have come to associate with 'normal adolescence'.

Davis (1990), in his historical exploration of the condition of youth in Britain, argues that the age-grade of adolescence as a theoretical entity was established for the first time in the late eighteenth-century writings of the French philosopher and writer Jean-Jacques Rousseau. In his conceptualisation of the ideal boy ('Emile'), Rousseau is said to have laid the foundation for an idea of a life-cycle divided into stages, each stage having its own physiology and set of tasks to be accomplished. He envisaged boyhood as a time of outdoor play, in which the boy was free to roam outside in loose clothing in what was seen as his 'natural' state. Formal education should not begin until the boy reached twelve years of age. Puberty was presented as marking a major shift from the carefree time of boyhood, bringing with it the 'tumultuous change' of adolescence and new birth into manhood. Rousseau expressed this forcefully, 'We are born, so to speak, twice over, born into existence and born into life; born a human being, and born a man' (quoted in Davis 1990: 41). Adolescence was innately and inevitably troublesome and stormy, requiring correct handling 'in order to ensure the smooth development of the individual and the continuity of society as a whole' (ibid.). Rousseau recommended that each adolescent boy should have his own personal tutor to give him careful instruction and guidance, unlikely to be an attainable goal for any but the most wealthy of families.

Interestingly, Rousseau was not only responsible for laying down the parameters of male adolescence. In writing about the ideal boy, 'Emile', he also wrote about the ideal girl, 'Sophie'. Unlike Emile, Sophie was to be trained in the home from an early age into domesticity and motherhood. This was, according to Rousseau, her 'natural' state. Gittins observes that in this depiction, Rousseau was 'naturalising' difference between the male world of the outdoor/public space and the female world of the indoor/private one (1998: 152).

If Rousseau was responsible for making adolescence a theoretical possibility, it was the social and economic changes that took place in the nineteenth century that made adolescence a practical reality for an increasingly broad cross-section of society. Gillis (1981) indicates that the eighteenth century had witnessed a steady growth in education for children of the upper and middle classes. A drop in child mortality amongst the aristocracy and middle classes meant that children growing up in smaller families found themselves spending more and more of their lives in controlled environments, at home and at school. Girls were most often kept at home until marriage, while middle and upper class boys stayed on longer at boarding schools. While older wage-earning working-class young people experienced a greater degree of freedom from parental control than before, others found themselves dependent for longer on their parents, as apprenticeships declined and secondary schooling increased.

Gillis argues that the reform of the elite public school consolidated the special character of adolescence. In the 1820s and 1830s, Thomas Arnold as headteacher introduced a new style of educational management to Rugby School, a style that was to be duplicated at public schools throughout the UK. Arnold instigated a military-style regime that envisaged the public school as a total institution in which the masters had a firm grip over all aspects of the boys' lives, educational and social. Gone were the days when the boys were free to spend their days as they chose, attending classes and instruction for only two or three hours a day. Now the boys' lives were to be structured into different phases of organised activity; games and sport were seen as a central part of this institutional framework. Gillis identifies in this the formation of a new cult of heterosexual masculinity in which physical strength, playing the game and sport were applauded as virtues, while femininity (and homosexuality) were associated with weakness and emotion.

There was, however, a quite different set of influences that contributed to the formation of the discourse around adolescence. Davis (1990) argues that there have been 'cycles of anxiety' in the parent culture around the issue of what might be termed 'juvenile delinquency' from at least the sixteenth century onwards (see also Pearson 1983). The late nineteenth and early twentieth centuries witnessed one such explosion of public concern about the behaviour of young people in the United States and across Europe. Davis (1990) points out that while the 'official model' of adolescence was being developed amongst upper- and middle-class children in the public and grammar schools, urban working-class young people had been developing their own distinctive subcultures. They had a higher degree of social and economic independence than ever before, their own entertainment (public house, football ground and music hall) and their own style of dress. There was universal fear and antagonism towards these so-called 'hooligans' or 'juvenile delinquents', illustrated in press and government statements of the day. Concern for the behaviour of young people came to a head in 1904 in the publication by American psychologist, G. Stanley Hall, of a massive two-volume work entitled *Adolescence, its Psychology and its Relation to Physiology, Anthropology, Sociology, Sex, Crime, Religion and Education*, widely read on both sides of the Atlantic. Here Hall took Rousseau's ideas about human development and about the special importance of a 'second birth' at puberty and reworked these in the light of post-Darwinian biology and evolutionist philosophy (Davis 1990: 60). He divided the life-cycle into four pre-adult developmental stages: 'infancy' (from birth to aged four years), 'childhood' (four to eight years), 'youth' (eight to twelve years), and 'adolescence' (puberty to adulthood). It was Hall, asserts Davis, who elevated the characteristic of 'storm and stress' to a central position within the psychology of the adolescent (1990: 61). (This issue will be explored further, see pp.93–5.)

Cross-cultural evidence

Studies of different cultures have pointed to the specificity of modern Western notions of youth and adolescence. For example, anthropologist Margaret Mead spent nine months in the 1920s living with young women in Samoa, observing their behaviour and their interactions with others: boys, elders and younger children. Her objective was to answer the question: 'Are the disturbances which vex our adolescents due to the nature of adolescence itself or to the civilization? Under different conditions, does adolescence present a different picture?' (1928: 17). Mead's resultant portrayal of Samoan life has been criticised for being rather idealised and idyllic; she is said to make uncritical assumptions about both Samoan and American adolescence (Springhall 1986). Nevertheless, her findings are of interest. She presents evidence that there were no differences between girls before and after puberty, except in relation to bodily changes. She asserts, therefore, that adolescence in Samoa was not characterised by any of the role confusion, conflict or rebellion which we take for granted as features of adolescence. Mead goes on to argue that explanations for youth rebellion and conflict must be sought in Western society and its organisation and age-structure (specifically, in a society that has too many choices and conflicting standards) instead of in young people or adolescence *per se.*

Banton's (1965) exploration of rites of passage in tribal societies also provides information about different patterns for understanding and organising the stage between childhood to adulthood. Banton points out that the period between childhood and adulthood can be a very short one in tribal societies, marked out by highly structured cere-monies and initiation customs. For example, he describes the initiation process that took place amongst the tribespeople in Sierra Leone in which young boys were taken out into the bush and given a series of tasks to accomplish over weeks or months. When they were brought back to the village, they were reborn as adults, and in some societies they were even given new names as confirmation of their new status as adults. Girls went through an equivalent, though less prolonged initi-ation. Banton argues that ceremonies and initiation customs like these help individuals to change roles, thus reducing the possibility of role confusion or uncertainty. (The concept of role will be explored further later in the chapter.)

Summary

Historical and cultural analyses of the development of youth demon-strate that common-sense notions about youth and young people are inextricably linked to the social, economic and cultural conditions of the day. Hence youth may be a very long or a very short period, depending on the wider structural and organisational context. Adolescence was itself created by the particular social and economic conditions which prevailed at the end of the nineteenth century, condi-tions which led to changes in the organisation of employment and education, and the emergence of a new period of dependency for young people during their teenage years. Psychological discourses were to provide the ideological backcloth through which the creation of adolescence was given meaning and purpose.

Psychological perspectives on youth

Freudian explanations

I have described in the work of G. Stanley Hall the beginnings of a psychological conceptualisation of youth as adolescence. Social work theory and practice have been greatly influenced by both psychological and psychoanalytic ideas.

Austrian psychoanalyst Sigmund Freud (1856–1939) believed that human beings pass through a number of distinct stages of development, and that each stage is characterised by different driving forces or tensions. How these tensions are handled will have an impact on subsequent personality traits, although most of us are unaware of the 'psychic processes' that take place at the unconscious level (see Coleman 1990 and 1992, Knuttila 1996, Meyerson 1975). The stages are described as follows:

- The oral stage – from birth to about two years of age, during which time infants' mouths are the focal point of their satisfaction and comfort, and the breast and feeding form the centre of the child's world.
- The anal stage – at two years, when infants discover the pleasure of some control over their bowel movements and the 'elimination of waste'; toilet training becomes a major task and potential area of conflict.
- The phallic stage – from three to about five years of age, as children discover their sexuality. This is the so-called Oedipal stage, when boys and girls are said to learn what will be 'normal' sex roles and behaviour by repressing the Oedipal (sexual) urges that they have in relation to their parents.
- The latency stage – from the fifth or sixth year until puberty, there occurs a latency period during which the young person's energies are taken up with social and learning activities and psychic conflicts are temporarily laid to rest.
- The genital stage – beginning at puberty, there is a rapid recapitulation of the three earlier stages of emotional development (oral, anal and phallic), and the unresolved Oedipal situation re-emerges. The end result of this stage of struggle and conflict is the achievement of 'normal' sexual identity and adult personality; whether this is successful or not will depend on the outcome of the three earlier phases.

The genital (adolescent) stage is thus presented as a potentially dangerous time, fraught with risks and challenges. Coleman (1992) describes in detail the psychoanalytic view of adolescence. The upsurge of instincts at puberty is said to upset the psychic balance that had been achieved by the end of childhood, thus causing internal emotional upheaval and leading to a greatly increased vulnerability of the personality. This state of affairs is accompanied by two additional factors. First, the individual's awakening sexuality directs him or her to look outside the family for appropriate 'love objects', thus breaking emotional ties with parents that have existed since infancy (a process known as disengagement). Second, the vulnerability of the personality leads to the employment of psychological defences to cope with the instincts and anxiety, which are, to a greater or lesser extent, maladaptive. Regression and ambivalence are seen as further key elements in the adolescent process, both resulting in nonconformity and rebellion, and thus advancing the disengagement process (1992: 11–13).

From this perspective, crises in adolescence are normal and necessary, because out of this period of upset and conflict comes mature adulthood, that is, 'healthy' heterosexual relationships outside the family. Anna Freud (1937 and 1958) is central to this tradition. She goes so far as to propose that it should be considered 'abnormal' if a child 'kept a steady equilibrium during the adolescent period ... The adolescent manifestations come close to symptom formation of the neurotic, psychotic or dissocial order and emerge almost imperceptibly into ... almost all mental illnesses' (Freud 1958).

Research carried out over the last twenty years by psychologists and social psychologists presents a more circumspect picture of adolescence. Results of this research suggest that, although adolescence may be a time of psychological difficulty and 'storm and stress' for some young people, this is by no means the norm. A notable study of fourteen- and fifteen-year-olds carried out by Rutter and his colleagues (Rutter *et al.* 1976) on the Isle of Wight illustrates this. The study discovered that ten-year-olds, fourteen-year-olds and adults suffered from psychiatric disorders in roughly similar numbers; that a substantial number of those who experienced psychiatric problems in adolescence had had problems since childhood; that when psychiatric difficulties did emerge in adolescence, this was often in the context of other stressful factors in the environment, such as parents' marital difficulties; that only 20 per cent of teenagers in the study agreed with the statement 'I often feel miserable or depressed' (quoted in Coleman 1979: 12). Rutter *et al.* conclude that the psychiatric importance of adolescence has probably been overestimated in the past (Rutter *et al.* 1976).

Feminist sociologists have been at pains to point out that adolescence is a masculine construct. Hudson (1984) argues that all our images of the adolescent – 'the restless, searching youth, the Hamlet figure, the sower of wild oats, the tester of growing powers' – are masculine images (1984: 35). This means that girls who behave in what is seen as an adolescent fashion will be thought of as not only displaying a lack of maturity (since adolescence is dichotomous with maturity) but importantly as not feminine. Thus girls who act out what are commonly regarded as adolescent roles, using challenging, nonconforming behaviour, risk far stronger retribution and measures of control than boys who exhibit similar behaviour. Hudson asserts that this has serious consequences for young women, who are caught between stereotyped images of adolescence and femininity, and are judged by two incongruent sets of expectations. They are left feeling that whatever they do is always wrong; 'a correct impression', she concludes, 'since so often if they are fulfilling the expectations of femininity they will be disappointing those of adolescence, and vice versa' (1984: 53).

Social psychologists writing today acknowledge that there is widespread variability in young people's experience of adolescence; that there may be as many adolescences as there are adolescents. Coleman (1990, 1992) argues that empirical evidence demonstrates that too much individual variation exists for young people of the same chronological age to be classified together. Adolescence, he asserts, should be viewed as a transitional process rather than a stage or even a number of stages. This transition is influenced by both internal and external pressures, that is, outside pressures from peers, parents, teachers and wider society, as much as from inside physiological and emotional pressures.

Developmental explanations

Alongside psychoanalytic interpretations, other psychological perspectives have explored human development in terms of stages of cognitive development (e.g. Piaget), moral development (e.g. Kohlberg), and identity development (e.g. Erikson).

Erik Erikson (1968) proposed a series of eight psychosocial stages to describe development from birth to death (the 'Eight Ages of Man'), based on the individual's ability to resolve a series of psychosocial crises and to establish appropriate social relations at each of these life stages (see Black and Cottrell 1993). Identity development was for Erikson a process of differentiation, as the separate self learns to accommodate increasing numbers of significant others. Erikson's stages are outlined as follows:

1st year – Trust versus mistrust.
2nd year – Autonomy versus shame and doubt.
3rd to 5th year – Initiative versus guilt.
6th year to puberty – industry versus inferiority.

Adolescence – Identity versus confusion.
Early adulthood – Intimacy versus isolation.
Middle adulthood – Generativity versus self-absorption.
Ageing years – Integrity versus despair.

Erikson affirms the idea that inner turbulence and identity problems are central features of the adolescent stage – young people are uncertain about who they are, and what they will do with their lives. He describes adolescence as a period of 'psychosocial moratorium': a time of enforced role-playing and experimentation during which conflicts and contradictions of identity must be resolved. The primary developmental crisis in adolescence is presented as a quest for identity: adolescence is about preparing for adult identity.

Springhall (1986) points out that there is little real social scientific evidence that any but a small minority of those in their teenage years experience a serious identity crisis, though there is clearly some change in the concept of self-identity at this time (1986: 227). Feminist psychologists have challenged the whole basis on which Erikson's analysis is built. Gilligan (1982) points out that Erikson's original research subjects were all men and boys, so that male behaviour and attitudes became the standard on which his developmental theory was based. When Erikson did conduct research on women, he discovered that their life-cycle was different to men's: women did not seek independence and differentiation as their ultimate goal in the way that men did, and instead expressed a desire to remain in association with others. Erikson analysed this gender difference by stating that male identity is forged in relation to the world, while female identity is awakened in a relationship of intimacy with another person, so that during adolescence, men and women have different tasks to accomplish. Whether or not this is the case, the underlying message was clear: full maturity was conceptualised as independence and differentiation (i.e. stereotypically male qualities). Gilligan argues that this has led to an ill-placed esteem for ideas of growth and independence, and a denigration of the values of integration and dependency.

Erikson's work has also been criticised by sociologists concerned to dispel the notion that there is something called 'normal' development. Wallace (1987) claims that in the psychology of adolescence, there has been an idea of a 'universal' developmental model of 'normal' transition: that is, adolescence means getting a job; having a hedonistic period of leisure and freedom; then 'settling down' to get married and moving into one's own house. But, Wallace argues, such transitions are not universal, for they differ according to 'race', sex and class, and this is related to the patterns of entry into work for different groups. Wallace states that at the time of her study (1986), young people in semi- and unskilled manual categories married an average of four years younger than those in professional and intermediate categories; similarly girls married three years earlier than boys. What this demonstrates is that transitions into work and family are variable; the transition from childhood dependence to independence from parents take place in different ways for different social groups at different periods of time. More recent studies of the impact of unemployment on young people's transitions (for example, MacDonald 1997) reinforce this complex picture. (The idea of transitions is discussed more fully later on pp. 111–14.)

Black perspectives on human development also call into question the usefulness of traditional psychological explanations. Robinson (1997) is unambiguous in her criticism of the Western psychological tradition. She writes:

The conventionally accepted paradigms and discoveries of Western psychology do not provide an understanding of black adolescents. Even a casual observation of the history of psychology will demonstrate that psychological literature over the last 100 years has been based on observations primarily on Europeans, predominantly male and overwhelmingly middle-class ... Despite the diversity of the various schools of Western psychology, they seem to merge unequivocally in their assumption of the Eurocentric point of view and the superiority of people of European descent. It is not surprising, therefore, that the conclusions reached are invariably of the inferiority of non-European peoples.

(1997: 152)

Robinson (1995 and 1997) argues that nigrescence (literally, 'the process of becoming black' or more concisely, the development of a black racial identity) is more relevant to black young people than conventional psychological theories on child development. She points out that several models of black identity development were introduced in the 1960s and 1970s. Each characterised identity development as a series of sequential stages, in which changes are influenced by an individual's reaction to social and environmental pressures and circumstances (1995: 100). Robinson suggests that Cross's (1971) model of the conversion from Negro to black is the most well known, and has been adapted by subsequent writers to make sense of the experience of a wide range of minority groups. Cross's five stages as detailed by Robinson are as follows (Robinson 1995: 101–3):

1   Pre-encounter – the person views the world from a white, Eurocentric frame of reference.
2   Encounter – a shocking event, personal or social, awakens the person to new views of being black and of the world.
3   Immersion–Emersion – the person struggles to destroy his or her former view of the world, immersing him or herself in blackness. (Cross, 1991, later writes that this stage can result in fixation and stagnation rather than identity development.)
4   Internalisation – the person achieves self-confidence with being black, and can now focus on things other than him/herself and his/her racial group.
5   Internalisation–Commitment – the person finds activities and commitments to express his or her new identity.

Tizard and Phoenix's (1993) study of young people of mixed parentage reviews the evidence for identity confusion amongst black and mixed-race children, and presents findings from their own research study of fifty-eight young people whose parents were both black and white. They report that early studies carried out in the late 1940s did indeed show a disturbingly high level of identity confusion amongst black children, who repeatedly misidentified themselves as white, and attributed 'bad' characteristics to black dolls in experiments. Subsequent studies have shown changes, however, and black children are now more likely to present positive self-images. Tizard and Phoenix's research demonstrated that 60 per cent of the mixed-parentage young people interviewed had a positive racial identity; 20 per cent had a problematic identity; and another 20 per cent were in an intermediate category, not definitely positive about their racial identity. They summarise their findings by suggesting that it is difficult to make generalisations about young people and identity. Class differences, gender differences, different schooling and different family backgrounds make for very different experiences for the young people concerned. This means that the experience of girls in a predominantly white middle-class school, protected from racism, were at complete odds with the experiences of working-class boys growing up in mixed communities, where both racism and a strong black culture were part of their day-to-day environment.

Implications for practice

Although I have argued that youth and adolescence are best understood as social constructions, this does not imply that the concepts have no resonance in the lives of young people. On the contrary, these concepts have a major influence both on young people themselves and on society as a whole. Young people may internalise and at the same time challenge ideas about what is normal and acceptable youthful conduct as they negotiate their journey into adulthood. Social work agencies today portray quite ambivalent views about youth, promoting conventional (and often conservative) notions about youth and adolescence, while at the same time forefronting young people's rights to self-determination.

A critical review of the psychological literature suggests that, although Freudian and developmental explanations undoubtedly contribute to social work's understanding of young people, social and societal explanations must also be taken into consideration. 'Adolescence' as a category was created by specific structural and economic factors; it is not a given, for all time. As a consequence, experiences of adolescence change across time and across groups of young people; adolescence is not necessarily the time of 'storm and stress' we have come to imagine it to be. While conventional psychological approaches may not offer sufficient understanding of the different experiences of young people, new feminist and black perspectives in psychology offer useful alternative frameworks for analysis.

Sociological approaches to youth

Sociological approaches stress the primacy of *social* understandings of young people's experience of youth. The focus is not on the individual's instincts, physiology or personality development, but on the social world in which the young person is growing up: the family, school, peer group and community, and at a broader level, society and its structured inequalities. Marsland (1987) makes a distinction between early sociological approaches – what he calls 'the conventional sociology of youth' – and later 'proto-Marxist' analyses. Conventional sociology between the 1950s and 1970s sought to understand youth as a social category, exploring such topics as role, peer group, generational conflict, and youth culture (for example, Banton 1965, Musgrave 1972). Later Marxist perspectives dismissed the concept of youth as an entity, and forefronted class as the dominant feature in the lives of young people (for example, Hall and Jefferson 1976, Willis 1977), while feminist sociologists highlighted the absence of girls in the youth studies (see Lees 1986, McRobbie and Garber 1976). Current sociological approaches to youth are concerned to understand the complex interconnections between age, class, gender, 'race' and ethnicity and sexuality for young people living in 'postmodern' society (see Abbott and Wallace 1990, MacDonald 1997).

Conventional sociological approaches to an understanding of youth

Role theory

As Chapter 3 has suggested, a central concern of sociologists has been to understand the process by which maturing members of society incorporate specific societal expectations and come to take their place as adult members of that society. This is explained in terms of role theory in very different ways, by functionalist and interactionist sociologists. Functionalist sociologists from Durkheim onwards have assumed that individuals learn the contents of their culture and the normative expectations that define their social roles through socialisation: 'people become social by learning social roles' (Fulcher and Scott 1999: 129). Social roles are seen as institutionalised social relationships that are matters of constraint, rather than personal choice; we largely accept the ways that roles have been defined and act accordingly. It is when we do not know how to behave, when roles are unclear or ill-defined, that individuals become unhappy and society begins to lose its cohesiveness.[1] Banton's (1965) analysis of the impact of changing roles on youth in industrial and pre-industrial societies illustrates a functionalist approach to role-theory.

Banton (1965) argues that moving from one role to another is not easy in complex industrial societies. Changing roles requires knowing the rights and obligations of the role and changes in behaviour; it also requires other people to recognise that a change in role has taken place and to modify their behaviour in a corresponding fashion. Peasant societies, Banton suggests, have few role changes, and have useful initiation ceremonies to mark the changes. In contrast, in industrial societies, there are no clear dividing lines between the roles of infant, juvenile and adult. This leads to strains on young people, who may look and feel physically mature, but are treated like children by their parents. Lengthening education, Banton argues, has exacerbated this discrepancy. Also, since knowledge is changing so fast, children may no longer see their parents are helpful role-models, or as even having a good enough understanding of the present world to be able to advise them, so that children have different, competing and unclear norms of behaviour to follow. Banton concludes that there is no clear dividing line between childhood and adulthood in modern societies, since children may well attend their parents' graduation ceremonies.

Banton's work made a significant contribution to shifting the focus of attention in the study of youth from individual, psychological concerns to events and structures in wider society. However, there has been substantial criticism of the idealised picture he presented of industrial and pre-industrial societies, and of the rather static presentation of the ways that roles operate in society. Interactionist sociologists present a more dynamic approach to understanding roles, arguing that at any one time, we play a number of different roles, and we make choices about how we will play or act out these roles (see Goffman 1969, Mead 1934). This would suggest that there is no 'essential' problem with role for young people. Various concepts have been developed from role theory: 'role-set' (the collection of many different roles that each of us plays); 'role conflict' (when one role competes with another, for example our role as employee and our role as parent), and 'role-distance' (when we choose to play a role but disengage from it while we are doing so).

Peer group

Much of the sociological writing on youth from the 1950s to the 1970s assumes that the peer group has increasing importance to young people. Musgrave (1972) defines the peer group as 'a homogeneous age group', and argues that in such a grouping, young people can gain experiences that would not be possible within the confines of the nuclear family. They are free to experiment, to have fun and to make mistakes, and most importantly, to practise relationships with members of the opposite sex. Smith describes this as 'the traditional, essentially structural-functionalist view of the influence of peers' (1987: 42). Peers are said to have an influence on socialisation in the spaces left by other institutions (principally the family and the school). The peer group is valued as a positive force, a place that provides support, security, understanding, and a sense of belonging. This in turn is fostered by the commercial exploitation of teenage purchasing power.

Smith (1987) distinguishes between a sociological literature that explores predominantly middle-class adolescents' peer groups and the criminological literature on juvenile delinquency, in which working-class peer groups are represented as 'gangs'. He criticises the presentation of young people in this writing, where peer groups are frequently portrayed as anti-school, anti-parent, or both (1987: 47). Smith argues from his own research that not all peer groups, and not all members of peer groups even amongst the working class, are anti-school. Smith is critical too of the absences in sociological investigation of peer groups – specifically the absence of girls and black young people. He draws attention to studies which suggest that working-class girls' peer groups may be qualitatively different to those of boys. He pinpoints criminological studies that illustrate the ways in which girls' peer groups may reinforce passivity, dependence and compliance among their members, whilst boys' groups are said to do quite the opposite (1987: 56).

McRobbie's research on girls' subcultures (McRobbie and Garber 1976) found strong supportive networks of friends amongst girls, and a real sense of solidarity between girls and their friends (1976: 143). Her findings have been echoed in more recent ethnographical research on girls' friendships, which describes these friendships as characterised by trust and loyalty. Griffiths (1995: 171) argues that friendships between women are a major way in which girls 'maintain some degree of power and control over their lives in a society in which women still occupy a subordinate position'. Griffiths also identifies conspicuous variations in the pattern of young women's friendships, so that they may be members of different groupings at school and at home. The school-based groups are likely to be single sex, close-knit groups of pairs or more, whilst neighbourhood groups tend to be larger, and less clearly differentiated in terms of age, 'race' or gender. This research suggests that we cannot make simple inferences based on the idea of 'a peer group', since young people are members of different peer groups, which provide different functions in their lives.

Generation gap

A third theme in the early sociological writing is the notion of a 'generation gap' between adults and young people. It is argued that the peer group is extremely important for young people who are thrown together for ever-longer periods with their own age group and largely segregated from adults. They share experiences, circumstances and problems which separate them from the outside world (see Eisenstadt 1956).

Social psychologist Rutter's study (see Rutter *et al.*, discussed on p.94) challenges the notion that alienation from parents during the teenage years is the norm. Researchers found that parents continue to have substantial influence over the opinions and behaviour of most young people. Hudson (1984) supports this analysis. She highlights studies which demonstrate that teenagers generally choose friends whose values are similar to, rather than in opposition to, those of their parents'. In her own study of fifteen-year-old girls, she found that most of those interviewed said that they generally agreed with their parents, and that disagreements were usually about trivial matters. She warns, however, that a discourse of adolescence framed in ideas of trouble and conflict leads parents, teachers and social workers constantly to expect trouble. More recent evidence from the Young People's Social Attitudes Survey conducted in 1994 confirms that young people's beliefs are not as radical as might be anticipated.[2] Newman (1996) claims that children and young people are not yet storming the bastions of adult power:

> They want parents to have a bigger say than themselves in the educational curriculum, they feel that drug use at school should be punished severely, they don't believe people should get married at a young age, leave school too early, or have sex below the current age of consent, and almost a third support current film censorship laws.
>
> (1996: 17)

Generation gap or culture clash?

While the relationship between white children and their parents has often been described in terms of a generation gap, the relationship between black children and their parents has frequently been analysed as a 'culture clash': black children challenging what are presented as the outdated customs and values of their parents. Brittan and Maynard (1984) see this perspective as implicitly racist: that is, a denigration of black culture. They assert that the focus should properly be on inter-generational conflict; on a rebellious period which any young person may go through, whether black or white.

Apter's (1990) research into relationships between black daughters and their parents makes a different point here. She demonstrates that neither generation gaps nor culture clashes are necessarily essential features of so-called 'second generation' black families. She demonstrates that authoritarian parents with a strong sense of their own culture do not, as has been suggested, raise less self-confident or dependent girls. Instead they raise self-assertive, competent girls.

Herbert (1997) reviews the evidence for a generation gap and finds it unconvincing. He maintains that, if anything, the generations are drawing together rather than apart. Young people tend to agree with their parents on the important issues (specifically moral and political issues) more than do parents and their parents (grandparents); the family continues to be of critical importance to young people, though of course there may be differences of opinion over minor issues such as dress and hair-style (1997: 90). Current research on culture suggests that ideas of a generation gap or culture clash may have even less meaning in the 1990s than previously, as the commercial leisure and fashion industry targets parents and young people alike as buyers of their products, whether this is music, clothing, food or films (see Jenks 1996).

Youth, youth culture and youth subcultures

Underpinning the functionalist sociological writing on youth in the years following the Second World War is the belief that youth and youth culture were both somehow qualitatively new and different from before. Youth is treated as if it were a 'new class' (Musgrove 1968). At the same time, ideas of 'postwar consensus', 'the affluent society', 'teenage consumers' and a new 'classless', meritocratic society contributed to the presentation of youth culture as a single, homogeneous culture, transcending all other cultural attachments of home, neighbourhood and class.

Osgerby (1998) asserts that the Second World War marked a crucial turning point in the development of British youth culture (1998: 17). In the decades that followed, a range of factors combined to highlight the visibility of the young as a distinct cultural entity:

- the postwar 'baby boom', which saw the youth population in the 1950s and 1960s grow;
- the Education Act of 1944, which raised the school leaving age to fifteen years and led to an increase of young people attending age-specific institutions and awaiting entry to the adult world of full-time employment;
- the expansion of the youth service and the rise of 'myriad attempts to marshal the leisure time of the young' (1998: 19);

- the introduction of National Service in 1948, which created a generation of young people caught in an 'interregnum' between leaving school and being 'called up' for two years at eighteen years of age (1998: 21);[3]
- the increased demand for the labour of young people and with it, the increased spending power of youth;
- the rise of mass communications – notably television – which promoted youth culture.

Davis (1990) argues that the period's preoccupation with youth was essentially an ambivalent phenomenon. Youth culture was at times portrayed in positive terms: young people were held up as the future of the nation, bright, bold and independent. Youth was 'the great national resource which if correctly and sufficiently utilized could still provide the way out of the nation's troubles' (1990: 208). But youth was also, at times, a negative, hostile presence – 'a portent of worse things to come' (ibid.) – and a symbol of all that was problematic about postwar society. Davis' own assessment is that it is the negative image of youth which has proved to have most resilience in the public imagination.[4]

The development of a radical analysis

Social class and youth

Perhaps the central point of disagreement between sociologists concerned with the study of youth has been the debate about the continuing centrality of social class. Functionalist sociologists (such as Parsons) believed that the new youth culture transcended class. Marxist scholars disagreed, arguing that youth culture could only be understood as reflecting wider (parental) class structures in society. Willis' study of working-class boys' attitudes to school provides a classic example of this perspective. Willis (1977) asserted that the lads' counter-school culture, although markedly at odds with the middle-class values of school, had a great deal in common with the working-class 'shop-floor' culture they would soon join as adult labourers. Their counter-culture in effect mirrored and anticipated working-class culture. Other studies have found that there are many similarities between working-class youth and parent cultures (for example, Humphries 1981) and that the differences between them have been exaggerated.

The work of the Centre for Contemporary Cultural Studies (CCCS) at the University of Birmingham has been highly influential in exploring youth and youth culture within a class analysis (see Hall and Jefferson 1976). CCCS researchers have been criticised for concentrating on the exotic and seemingly glamorous aspects of male working-class youth subcultures, and for failing to examine their negative aspects, or the personal responsibility which young people have for their actions (Hill and Tisdall 1997). Nevertheless, the importance of the work of the Centre should not be understated. In *Resistance through Rituals*, Clark *et al.* (1976) present a carefully considered historical analysis of the connections between ideas of class, youth culture and youth subcultures. They argue that the 'rediscovery' of poverty and continuing inequalities of wealth in the 1960s demonstrate that class and class conflict continue to have meaning in society. Leading on from this, they propose that the idea of a homogeneous youth culture is an illusion and a 'social myth'. They write:

> what it disguises and represses – differences between different strata of youth, the class-basis of youth cultures, the relation of 'Youth Culture' to the parent culture and the dominant culture, etc. is more significant than what it reveals.
>
> (1976: 15)

Clarke *et al.* propose that 'youth culture' must be deconstructed and replaced with the term 'subculture', reflecting the connections between subcultures and class relations, the division of labour, and productive relations of the society (1976: 16). Further, they warn against making assumptions about subcultures. Subcultures, they argue, may come and go. Some are regular and persistent features of the 'parent' class culture; others appear only at particular historical moments – 'they become visible, are identified and labelled (either by themselves or by others): they command the stage of public attention for a time: then they fade, disappear or are so widely diffused that they lose their distinctiveness' (1976: 14). Individual young people, similarly, move in and out of one, or perhaps several subcultures; and the great majority of young people will not enter a coherent subculture at all. 'For the majority, school and work are more structurally significant – even at the level of consciousness – than style and music' (1976: 16). For those who are part of subcultures, however, the subculture has particular functions as a symbolic form of resistance to the economic rituals and upheavals of the postwar period:

Though not 'ideological', sub-cultures have an ideological dimension: and in the problematic situation of the post-war period, this ideological component became more prominent. In addressing the 'class problematic' of the particular strata from which they were drawn, the different sub-cultures provided for a section of working-class youth (mainly boys) *one* strategy for negotiating their collective existence. But their highly ritualised and stylised form suggests that they were also *attempts at a solution* to that problematic experience: a resolution which, because pitched largely at a symbolic level, was fated to fail. The problematic of a subordinate class experience can be 'lived through', negotiated or resisted; but it cannot be *resolved* at that level or by those means.

(1976: 47)

Numerous studies from the 1950s onwards have examined the behaviour and rituals of particular cultural formations of predominantly English working-class young men: teddy boys (1950s), mods and rockers (1960s), skinheads, punks and football hooligans (1970s and 1980s). In reviewing this literature, Garratt (1997) suggests that subcultures are probably 'nothing more than a means to create and establish an identity in a society where they [young people] can find it difficult to locate a sense of self' (1997: 143). Subcultures may seem to be a challenge to adult society, but this challenge is symbolic rather than real, since it is based on aesthetics and fashion. Subcultures, he argues, have a positive value to the individual and society: 'They give young people the chance to express their difference from society, yet co-exist within it' (1997: 149).

Girls in the study of youth

Feminist sociologists have highlighted the ways in which analyses of youth culture and subcultures serve to obscure the differences between young people, and more so, the power differentials between particular groups of young people, in this case, boys and girls.[5] In *Resistance through Rituals*, McRobbie and Garber (1976) claim that the absence of girls from the whole literature is striking – where young women do make an appearance, they are usually seen in ways that are marginal, or which reinforce a stereotyped image of women. They pose explanations for girls' absence and conclude that girls negotiate a different space to boys, and offer 'a different type of resistance to what can at least in part be viewed as their sexual subordination'. Girls form small self-supporting, insulated groups, which exclude others – 'undesirable' girls, boys, adults, teachers and researchers (1976: 221–2).

Nava (1984) and Lees (1986) similarly provide a strong denunciation of the neglect of girls in the study of youth. In her study of youth work, Nava asserts that the screening of power differentials leads boys to 'lay claim to the territory of the [youth] club, and inhibits attempts by girls to assert their independence from them' (1984: 13). It also makes more difficult the building of alliances between women youth-workers and girls, a situation which Nava suggests improved in the 1980s with the introduction of girls' groups in youth work, and the development of a new feminist youth work. Lees (1986) takes a different (but equally critical) approach, exploring the representation of young women's sexuality in 1960s and 1970s studies of youth culture. She points out that young women in (male) youth studies are presented in terms of their sexuality rather than as human beings: as 'slag' or 'drag', 'virgin' or 'whore'. This, she argues, is 'a crucial mechanism in ensuring their subordination to boys and men' (1986: 14–15). Girls are referred to as passive creatures, on the edges of, or marginal to boys' activity: 'girls flit in and out of the pages as sex objects in the boys' eyes' (1986: 16). Lees concludes that young people negotiate their sexuality and behaviour within powerful constraints; masculine and feminine behaviour is subject to different social rules and operates within different norms.

Youth culture, subcultures and delinquency

The sociological study of youth (whether focused on peer groups, cultures or subcultures) has been consistently framed in terms of an idea of young people as 'troublesome'. Young people are seen to pose a threat both to society and to the status quo.

In his historical analysis of street crime and hooliganism, Pearson (1983) points out that it is commonplace to look back nostalgically to a 'golden age' of order and security, often described as '20 years ago' or 'before the war' (both First and Second World Wars). This 'golden age' is held up as a period of peace and stability, with low levels of crime and high levels of popular respect for law and order. Pearson demonstrates that the notion of a tranquil past has no historical validity. On the contrary, documentary evidence suggests that there was widespread fear amongst the middle classes in the nineteenth century about working-class street crime, violence, vandalism, drunkenness and lack of respect for the police. In the 1850s and 1860s, this crystallised around the discovery of a 'new' street crime, called 'garrotting', in which the victim was choked and robbed. Pearson argues that the public reaction to 'garrotting' and an increase in policing led to the creation of a 'crime wave', much as the street crime of 'mugging' came to public attention in the 1970s (1983: 144).

Concerns about the behaviour of young people can be found as far back as Roman and Greek civilisations. Pearson charts the successive panics which have erupted in the UK about young people, from apprentices in the 1600s to 'hooligans' in the 1880s. He writes:

> Across the centuries we have seen the same rituals of territorial dominance, trials of strength, gang fights, mockery against elders and authorities, and antagonism towards 'outsiders' as typical focuses for youth energy and aggressive mischief. Even under vastly different social conditions there are striking continuities between the violent interruptions to pre-industrial fairs and festivals, and the customary eruptions during modern Bank Holidays or the weekly carnival of misrule at contemporary football games – where the modern football rowdy ... must seem like a reincarnation of the unruly apprentice or the late Victorian 'Hooligan'.
>
> (1983: 221)

Pearson goes on to ask why young people feature so heavily in criminal statistics. He concludes that biological explanations are not enough: they do not provide sufficient explanation for either crimes of violence themselves, nor for our preoccupation with them. He argues that the answer must instead be sought in ideology. The focus on young people, their leisure habits and pastimes at the end of the nineteenth century must, for Pearson, be understood as a concerted attack on working-class culture; as an attempt to control and contain the so-called 'dangerous classes'. The children of the urban poor epitomised the threat of proletarian revolution; they therefore needed to be educated and institutionalised into middle-class values.

Working-class young people have continued to be seen as a threat and a danger, as subsequent moral panics about their behaviour reveal. Cohen's classic study of 'Mods' and 'Rockers' (1972) describes a specific moment when social reaction to the behaviour of particular groups of young people encouraged them away from intermittent deviancy towards a firm commitment to a deviant career: they effectively took on the personae of their stereotyped labels. Cohen points out that working-class youngsters had traditionally visited seaside resorts at holiday times, but at Easter 1964 in Clacton, the weather was cold and wet and tempers frayed. There were scuffles between local youths and visiting Londoners, and some beach huts and windows were damaged. The press reaction was furious, and for the rest of that year and subsequent years in the 1960s, sensational press coverage accompanied disturbances at a number of British seaside resorts. Cohen demonstrates that media reaction played an active role in shaping events, leading to a 'deviancy amplification spiral' which consolidated and magnified the original behaviour (this theme will be developed in Chapter 7).

Sociologists in the 1980s and 1990s have argued that delinquency and social reaction to delinquent behaviour are rooted in gender and 'race' expectations as well as norms and assumptions based on class. Hudson (1988) asserts that people expect trouble from male youths: it is part of growing up and learning to be a man. Women in trouble, however, are constantly sexualised and their behaviour is interpreted on the basis of sexuality. Hudson expresses this as follows:

> What society expects of its white young men and views as normal behaviour is different more in degree than in kind from behaviour condemned as delinquent: these expectations contrast significantly with the agenda for young women who are expected to learn for a life of passivity, servitude and domesticity. Delinquency ... provides one means for developing an identity as a man.
>
> (1988: 37)

There are also found to be significant differences in the experiences of black young people living in the UK, so that behaviour tolerated from white youth may not be tolerated from black youth. Hudson states that there is considerable evidence that state agencies are likely to perceive black youth's behaviour as problematic and in need of some form of controlling intervention more quickly, and more intensively. She suggests that this may be related to the readiness of professionals to mis-recognise and pathologise the culture of Afro-Caribbean and Asian families (again, this theme will be developed in Chapter 7).

Current themes in the sociology of youth

Demographic and economic changes

Davis (1990) asserts that one of the major shifts we are witnessing in the UK as we move towards the twenty-first century is the dramatic change in the age-structure of the population. The birth-rate has been falling since a peak in 1964, and as numbers of young people have declined, so a higher proportion of youth is engaged in education and training. Davis predicts that the implications are that we will reach a situation where 'appropriately qualified young people are at a premium', while a significant unqualified minority will face persistent unemployment and deepening social problems (1990: 215).

In fact, the recession of the 1980s has meant that youth unemployment has reached far higher levels than might have been anticipated. Roberts (1995) records that in 1972, nearly two-thirds of young people left school at sixteen years of age and most entered full-time work almost immediately. In 1992, however, fewer than one in ten sixteen-year-olds entered employment directly from school. At the same time, increasing numbers of young people have either chosen to stay on at school, or have found themselves in some form of youth training scheme. These demographic and societal changes have had a major impact on youth transitions – that is, on the ways in which young people grow up and enter adulthood.

Youth transitions

Sociologists have been interested for many years in the idea of the transitions that young people make as they move into adulthood (see Hill and Tisdall,1997: 115):

• transitions from family of origin to adult sexual partnership(s);
• transitions from school to work;
• transitions from parental income to own income;
• transitions from family household to own household.

In the 1950s and 1960s, functionalist sociologists accepted that a 'normative transition' existed, one which all young people were said to make (that is, leave school, get a job, become engaged, get married, move into a new home). The transitions of specific individuals and groups could then be compared alongside this 'normal' transition. More recently, Marxist and feminist sociologists have pointed out that there is no such thing as a 'normal' transition. They have instead identified systematic variations in transitions, so that paths into adulthood may be longer or shorter, straightforward or more complex, depending on factors such as class, gender and ethnicity (see Abbott and Wallace 1990, Wallace 1987). Working-class boys, for example, were found to be more likely to have an 'accelerated' transition, attaining adult status relatively quickly after leaving school. In comparison, middle-class young people were more likely to go into higher education and post-pone entry to the world of work, hence 'protracting' their transitions.

There is general agreement in sociological writing today that transitions continue to be structured by factors such as social class, family background, gender, 'race', educational achievement and opportunities in the local labour market (see Abbott and Wallace 1990, Chisholm and Du Bois-Reymond 1993, Jones and Wallace 1992, Pilcher 1995). Recent research, however, demonstrates that transitions are even more varied than this, reflecting other, more personal issues. Banks *et al.*'s research (1992) on sixteen- to nineteen-year-olds in four British cities (Swindon, Liverpool and Sheffield in England, and Kirkcaldy in Scotland) uncovered widespread variation amongst the transitions of young people. While most young people did, as expected, undergo transitions that could be described as 'protracted', there were many different reasons for, and feelings about this experience. Some protracted transitions were said to be voluntary, others were enforced; some were thought to be positive, others negative. Experiences of boys and girls, although very similar while remaining in education, were markedly different afterwards, with boys and girls heading for very different segments of the labour market. Young women also made more extensive contributions to household labour, whatever their class, although this was accentuated in working-class families. This study thus brings back human 'agency' to transitions' research, suggesting that a structural analysis is not sufficient explanation in itself.

Debates about the nature of agency and structure in youth transitions continue to attend research into transitions. The question remains, how much freedom do young people have to make their own decisions regarding the transitions they make? Jones and Wallace in their analysis of transitions offer the following assessment:

> although the social structure of stratification based largely on class, gender, race and ethnic inequalities affects young people's life chances from birth, during their life course they steer their way, with varying degrees of success, through formal and informal institutional structures which put new constraints and opportunities in their paths.
>
> (1992: 142)

The actions of some young people, they advise, should by implication, be understood as 'informed choice strategies' arising from opportunity. Other actions are 'survival strategies' arising from constraint. Jones and Wallace are realistic about the overall nature of opportunity and constraint. They suggest that constraints outweigh opportunities in many more cases, with young people being channelled in training courses that are not of their choosing. They also claim that youth as a whole is disadvantaged by its lack of an organised voice or representation in trade unions and political parties. Nevertheless, they are insistent on the importance of studying the scope of individuals within structures. Rudd and Evans (1998) are also interested in individual agency. In their study of the aspirations of college students doing vocational courses, they discover high degrees of both optimism and realism amongst students. The students expect to get work – but not necessarily immediately or for all time. This suggests a very different attitude to employment from former ideas of the importance of securing 'a job for life'.

Irwin (1995) brings another insight into the analysis of youth transitions. She is critical of the pre-eminence given to explanations based on employment restructuring and the declining demand for youth labour in conventional transitions studies. She points out that any hypothesis of a deferral in the transition from dependence to independence entails a 'restructuring of the relations between dependants and those on whom they make claims for resources' (1995: 298). In other words, she urges that the transition to adulthood must be located in the context of wider social changes, including most crucially, the increasing importance of paid employment amongst women in the postwar decades. Women's paid work has allowed young adults to stay on in full-time education and take on relatively low-paid jobs. In addition, delays in household and family formation by young people are at least in part a reflection of the increased importance of young women's earnings.

Pilcher (1995) agrees that we should be cautious about explaining changes in transitions solely in terms of employment changes. She reminds us that courtship behaviour and patterns of marriage and childbirth have themselves undergone change since the 1970s. Young people are now more likely to leave home and share flats or houses with other young people before going on to set up households with a sexual partner. Changes in the labour market have not prevented young people from growing up and becoming adults, though changes in social security benefits have made it difficult for young people without employment to leave home and set up their own home.

Roberts (1997), in summarising the current state of knowledge on youth transitions, concludes that, in spite of dire warnings from sociologists about the probability of 'broken' and 'fractured' transitions, young people have coped surprisingly well: transitions have been 'restructured, rather than destroyed'. He gives three examples to demonstrate this viewpoint. First, he argues that large numbers of young people have coped with periods of unemployment, in some instances better than adults. Second, they have continued, on the whole, to be supported by their families. Third, they have adapted to their new roles as students and trainees. This is a much less pessimistic picture of young people today, and one which suggests that young people can, to a degree, influence their transitions. They are active agents in a wider context of structural, political and demographic change.

From classless to underclass

I have drawn attention above to the popular idea in the postwar years that Britain had entered a new 'classless' society and that youth and the 'affluent teenager' were at the forefront of this development. In recent years, the focus has been much less upbeat and optimistic. Youth has been portrayed in the media as a part of the 'underclass', separate from, and at the same time undermining society as a whole. Within the underclass discourse, key figures have been given particular prominence: the young single mother, the absent father, the unemployed black youth, the working-class housing estate. Sociologists (as we will consider) have been deeply divided about the existence, and the potential usefulness or dangerousness of the concept of underclass.

Roberts (1995 and 1997) represents sociological thinking which accepts the idea of underclass and believes it is visible in the UK today. Roberts defines an underclass as follows (1997: 42–3):

1   The stratum should be disadvantaged relative to, and in this sense beneath, the lowest class in the gainfully employed population.
2   For the individuals and households involved this situation should be persistent, in many cases for the duration of their entire lives and, indeed, across the generations.
3   The underclass should be separate from other groups in social and cultural respects as well as in its lack of regular employment. For example, its members might live in separate areas, belong to separate social networks, and have distinctive lifestyles and values.
4   The culture of the underclass ... should have become another impediment, and sufficient in itself even if other obstacles were removed, to significantly reduce its members' likelihood of joining the regularly employed workforce.

Roberts (1995) argues that there are clear strands of evidence of under-class formation in Britain which cannot be ignored. He identifies these as follows (1995: 101–4):

- Long-term unemployment is common amongst certain groups.
- Some young people do lose contact with mainstream social institutions and become invisible to official data collection, for example, homeless young people.
- Some young people are unlikely to be recruited by any employer, because of their limited physical or mental abilities or persistent drug use.
- Some young people do opt out into subcultural groupings: stealing and hustling become a way of life to them.
- Finally, cycles do tend to repeat themselves: people with disadvantaged family origins tend to have children who repeat the cycle with their own children.

Roberts takes issue with British sociology's resistance to underclass theory, arguing that this opposition is at least in part ideological. British sociologists, he declares, have a vested interest in sustaining an orthodox social class framework that is not weakened by any notion of a class existing underneath the working class. However, this viewpoint is challenged by recent sociological writing which rejects the notion of an underclass as both unconvincing as a structural explanation and personally stigmatising for those who are labelled as underclass.

The contributors to MacDonald's (1997) edited collection present a robust critique of underclass theory. They point to the ways in which young people have been excluded from society, marginalised from economic structures and shut out from any feeling of social citizenship: far from choosing to opt out to live on benefits, the opportunities for them to join society have been progressively diminished. Baldwin, Coles and Mitchell (1997) argue that underclass theories over-simplify the complex processes of social exclusion which lead heterogeneous groups of vulnerable young people (such as care leavers and those with special needs and disabilities) along unsuccessful transitions. Others argue for more coherent social policies which recognise the dangerousness of underclass ideas. In writing about young people and housing, Jones (1997) proposes that we need to replace right-wing representations of an underclass with a more sociological analysis of the interplay of structure and agency in shaping the risky housing transitions of youth.

The return of youth subculture

The 1990s have witnessed a new flowering of youth cultural studies, focusing this time on the 'rave' phenomenon, deadhead culture and 'post-political pop' (Redhead 1990, Epstein 1998). As the dominance of 'common culture' breaks up, so 'style' and subculture are again presented as ways in which young people cope with their worlds. But now their worlds are fragmented, pluralist and individualistic, that is, thoroughly postmodern. Willis (1990) describes this as follows:

> The strengthening, emerging, profane common culture is plural and decentred but nevertheless marks a kind of historical watershed. There is now a whole social and cultural medium of inter-webbing common meaning and identity-making which blunts, deflects, minces up or transforms outside or top-down communication. In particular, 'elite' or 'official' culture has lost its dominance − the very sense, or pretence, of a national, whole culture and of hierarchies of values, activities and places within it is breaking down.
>
> (1990: 128)

But there is another trend pulling in the opposite direction, that is, the globalisation of culture. This means that, at the same time as young people's lives are becoming more varied, so they are also becoming more homogeneous. Stewart (1992) argues that one of the most powerful influences cementing the 'shared' experience of young consumers has been the pervasiveness of American cultural norms and commercial brands:

> American brands such as Coke and Levis, or cultural icons such as Michael Jackson or Madonna, have established an almost universal appeal among young people the world over, to such as extent that they have become synonymous with youth and fully integrated into the mainstream culture.
>
> (1992: 224)

Summary

The breadth and depth of the sociological studies discussed have clearly demonstrated the importance of a sociological understanding of youth. The picture that emerges in the sociology of youth is predominantly one of tension: tension between parental culture and youth culture, between continuity and change, between shared understandings and diversity and difference. Young people inhabit the same structural position in terms of age. Beyond this point, there is no homogeneous 'youth' and no single 'youth culture'. On the contrary, factors such as class, gender, 'race' and ethnicity, sexuality and disability have a profound impact on the life chances and situations of young people. Economic changes since the 1980s have seriously undermined the patterns of employment for young people and extended the period of their dependency. At the same time, changes in social attitudes have meant that family and relationship patterns have altered too. Young people are not necessarily the delinquent, dangerous, troublesome underclass portrayed in the tabloid press. But at the same time, numbers of young people are systematically excluded from society – from education, employment, housing and mainstream society. They have become the scapegoats of society, just as young people have been society's scapegoats in the past (see Pearson 1983).

Implications for practice

The need for a sociological insight into youth is unequivocal. Social workers most frequently work with those who have been disadvantaged in society: the poor, the working-class, the young, the old, those with disabilities. It is crucial that in working with young people, social workers have an understanding of the structural basis of disadvantage and inequality, taking into account the continuing impact of changes in employment, social security and educational systems as well as the influence of structural factors such as class, age, 'race' and ethnicity, gender and sexuality.

Young people today throughout the world have little access to power and to resources. In the UK, the 1990s has seen a gradual erosion of welfare benefits (housing and income benefits) available to young people, just as student grants have been drastically cut. The sight of young people begging on the streets of our cities no longer merits public attention: it has become a fact of life. At the same time the provision of preventive services for young people and families has been reduced: family centres and youth clubs have closed as local authorities struggle to cope with financial restraints. Social work services have increasingly been targeted at attempting to monitor and control children and young people deemed to be 'at risk' (Hallett 1993), rather than meeting any broader imperative to counteract social inequality or in the words of the Social Work (Scotland) Act of 1968 to 'promote social welfare'. This is a situation that individual social workers must seek to change, in partnership with service-users, if we are not going to see the 'failure of the profession' that Jones (1997) predicts in the title of his recent article.

Conclusion

This chapter began by suggesting that young people have typically been regarded as a social problem: the 'troubled' and 'troublesome' of psychological and sociological literature. The reality is much more complex and contradictory. The social category of 'youth' is in practice created, and at the same time contested, by the very discourses (the ideas and practices) which set its boundaries. Beyond this, the experience of young people is immensely variable. Differences between young people are structured into society (through gender, class, sexuality, disability and 'race') as well as being specific to individuals' biographies, histories and personalities. Continuities and connections between adult and youth cultures must be understood alongside the changes and disruptions which both adults and youth experience.

Out of all the literature and research discussed in this chapter, two specific ideas have particular resonance for social work. The first is that we sometimes expect trouble from young people simply because that is the way the discourses around youth and adolescence are framed (Hudson 1984). Second, what young people want from us is a bigger say in the way their lives are run (Newman 1996). Taken together, these ideas provide a way forward for policy and practice.

Recommended reading

- Coleman, J.C. (1990) *The Nature of Adolescence*, Second edition, London: Routledge (reviews the psychological and social psychological literature).

- Jones, H. (ed.) (1997) *Towards a Classless Society?*, London: Routledge (an interesting edited collection which is mainly concerned with youth and young people).
- MacDonald, R. (ed.) (1997) *Youth, the 'Underclass' and Social Exclusion*, London: Routledge (an zedited collection from a radical perspective).
- Osgerby, B. (1998) *Youth in Britain since 1945*, Oxford: Blackwell (a good historical account).

5 Community

Introduction

This chapter and the next one should be read in conjunction with one another, since they both consider sociologically another key aspect of social work practice: community care. Community care social workers work in area teams, GP practices, hospitals and hospices with a wide range of service-users and their carers – older people, people with disabilities (both physical disabilities and learning disabilities), and people with mental health problems. Each user-group has its own individual issues that require specialist skills and knowledge, knowledge which is likely to draw on psychological and medical as well as sociological understanding. What brings these groups together, however, is the context in which they come to the attention of social work and social workers, that is, the context of community care. Chapters 5 and 6 are about that context: about the ways in which ideas of 'community' and 'caring' have influenced (and continue to influence) social work practice with older people, sick people, those with mental health problems and those with disabilities and their care-givers.

I have deliberately separated out the concepts of 'community' and 'caring' into two chapters so that each can be considered in its own right. This is necessary because so often literature about community care assumes that the two inevitably go together, as if we cannot have one without the other. I believe that community and caring are not essentially either indivisible or even the same entity, and that by always conceptualising them as one thing, we lose sight of the individual meanings of each and the possible contradictions between the two. It is vital for the development of sensitive, anti-discriminatory policy and practice in social work that we take a step back from community care as a 'catch-all' phenomenon, and instead forefront the views and experiences of care-recipients and care-givers in the planning and provision of services.

This chapter examines the concept of community, investigating the historical and sociological bases of community as the term exists in everyday usage and as it permeates social work policy and practice.

Definitions of community

In common with the notion of 'the family', the word 'community' carries with it a host of ideas and assumptions that are largely taken for granted. Most of the time, when we think of 'community', we do so in positive terms: it is something (again, like the family) which acts as a barrier to, or defence against, the stresses and ills of modern living. It is 'a good thing', something that we value and something that is frequently perceived as having declined in the shift to a modern, industrial, urban society. In order to make an objective assessment of this, we need to ask: what is community?

Sociologists have come up with very many different ways of describing community. In 1955, Hillery attempted to define community by examining its usage in sociological literature. He identified no fewer than ninety-four definitions, with little consensus between writers about what the concept meant. He claimed that 'beyond the recognition that "people are involved in community" there is little agreement on the use of the term' (1955: 117). More recent investigations have confirmed this conceptual confusion, with more than 200 identified definitions (McMillan and Chavis 1986). Although definitions vary in emphasis, they also share certain common features. There are broadly three ways of characterising community:

- Community as locality: community is defined as a physical–spatial entity; it is based on geographical location such as neighbourhood, village, town or place.
- Community as social network: a community is said to exist when a network of interrelationships is established between people who live in the same locality.
- Community as relationship (or 'communion'): community is defined as a shared sense of identity between individuals, irrespective of any local focus or physical proximity.

As we will discover, some sociologists in writing about communities have collapsed the three definitions into one, assuming that locality, social networks and shared identity are necessarily contingent on each other. Others have focused on one aspect, such as social networks, rejecting the usefulness of notions of locality or identity. In reality, communities are highly variable and complex, as this chapter will demonstrate. Physical localities may be places characterised by racism and exclusion of individuals and groups rather than networks of caring relationships or shared identities. Social networks may thrive across large geographical distances and may even be world-wide, facilitated by modern communication systems such as telephone, email and the Internet. In addition, shared identity may have little to do with location or even with local social networks. The sense of belonging which people feel may derive from their connectedness to a totally different country or culture to that of their local neighbourhood. As patterns of occupational mobility and migration increase, so this is likely to become more common. Bell and Newby (1976: 197) point out that there is a paradox here. As localism has declined as a structural principle – we no longer live, work and play in the same locality all our lives – so the idea of community (and our yearning for it) has grown.

Community discourses

It is clear from the discussion so far that when we think about community, we enter the realms of discourses and ideologies, that is, the ideas, beliefs, values and practices that characterise community, rather than any objective 'facts' about community. Symonds (1998) suggests that the concept of community occupies two parallel realities. The first is the 'social lived reality' in which people work and live, a reality that recognises conflicts and difference, and is aware that social networks are not always supportive and friendly. The second is the 'dream' world of community:

> This community 'in the mind' is always warm, supportive, safe and secure. This picture has been transmitted culturally through literature, certain historical 'readings', sociology, and in television soap operas. Interestingly the place of this dream community tends to be a small area inhabited by people who share the same culture, characteristics, history, language and understanding of their world.
>
> (1998: 12)

The 'community in the mind' may seem cosy and comfortable. In reality, it is a far from comfortable place for those who do not seem to fit this ideal 'dream'. Politicians and intellectuals in the United States and in the UK have used the idea of community to promote particular (and essentially conservative) views about family form and community life. Community in the sense of 'communitarianism' may seem, on the one hand, to be giving value to ideas of locality, neighbourliness and sharing. Seen in a different light, it may stigmatise some kinds of living arrangement, and lead to unrealistic expectations of community support that do not take sufficient account of structural inequalities in society (see Etzioni 1994, McIntosh 1996, Murray 1990).

Implications for practice

The discussion of definitions is important for policy and practice for two principal reasons. First, because the term is used very widely, it is not at all clear just what 'community' means in a given usage. We have community service, community homes, community workers, community development, community action, community programmes, community teams, and of course community care, and all may mean something quite different. The confusion and contradiction inherent in this must be acknowledged, because it can pull social work in totally opposite directions. This is evident in the tension between the urge to deprofessionalise social work, to make it a neighbourhood-based, co-operative activity (that is, community social work as envisaged by the 1982 Barclay Report) and the drive to assert social work's professional status through care management and the 1990 National Health Service and Community Care Act.

Second, social workers must be able to distinguish between community as 'normative prescription' (what the writer believes it should be) and 'empirical description' (what it actually is) (Allan 1991: 108). Hence it is always political, used by those on the Left to emphasise collective identity control/government at a localised level; and by those on the Right to symbolise freedom from dependence on the state, and individual choice and family responsibility.

In order to understand the impact of the 'dream' world of community on social work practice, we must first examine the historical and sociological writing on the concept of community.

Historical accounts

Conventional sociological perspectives are premised by the assumption that communities in the past were more vibrant, more secure and more caring than in the present. Certainly there have been huge social, economic and demographic changes over the past 200 years or so. Mills (1996) outlines the scale of changes that have taken place in Britain. The Industrial Revolution, conventionally defined as the period 1760 to 1830, led to the concentration of industrial activity on the coalfields and at the ports. Rural domestic industries declined rapidly, as did local self-sufficiency. The population of England and Wales doubled between 1700 and 1800, again between 1801 and 1851, and yet again between 1851 and 1911. Because much of the increased population was migrating to the towns in the nineteenth century, the population of most rural areas declined. As the rural population declined, so did agricultural employment. The massive growth in towns and cities provides the other side of the coin. The concentration of large populations in small areas led to many environmental and social problems. But, Mills argues, Victorian cities were more prosperous than any that had come before and were able to pay for amenities such as lighting, water sewerage, transport, dispensaries and universal schooling. New forms of transport within and outside the cities and towns encouraged the movement of people to and from the countryside, so that it became possible for rural workers to live in villages and travel to towns to work, just as town-dwellers moved out to live in new suburbs and villages on the edge of towns. Mills reports that the inversion of the social composition of a rural population took no more than fifty years, as middle-class town-dwellers replaced farm labourers or village craftsmen in the countryside. Alongside this shift, amenities and community welfare have declined in inner-city areas, although in some cities this trend has been halted by the upgrading ('gentrification') of some run-down areas to provide housing for single professional people. Mills concludes that community at the beginning of this period might be largely defined in terms of territory; today people live, shop, work and socialise in different territories and, he argues, in different communities (1996: 272–5).

This brief pen picture of social, economic and demographic change demonstrates that there has been a transformation in community as territory in Britain. But what can this tell us about the less tangible definitions of community, that is, about community as social networks or relationship? Dennis and Daniels (1996) indicate that because no agreement has been reached on indices of community life, it is difficult to assess if and how community life has changed over time. The relative value placed on the notion of social mix in a community illustrates this point. Some writers assume that a degree of social mixing is a prerequisite of community, so that community life declines as segregation intensifies. Others believe that because community is based on class, it is more likely to develop as segregation increases. In reviewing the evidence from historical documents, Dennis and Daniels point out that nineteenth-century sources can tell us where people lived and near whom, how often they moved, where they worked, to whom they were related and whom they married. 'But', they ask critically, 'do these findings have any value as evidence of community life?' (1996: 203).

Oral histories and autobiographies give us further insight into community life in the past. Many of these accounts stress the quality · of relationships between people, as poverty and hardship forced people to rely on each other for support. Many are also touched by the soft, rosy hues of nostalgia:

> In those days, too, there was real neighbourliness. You see, you might be four or five families in that house, and perhaps the one at the bottom would make some tea and she'd shout up the stairs 'I've just made a cup of tea – coming down?' And they'd more or less take it in turn each day, and if there was anyone in real dire straits, and couldn't pay their way, I've known a neighbour take their own sheets off the bed, wash 'em and pawn 'em to help them out. That's how it was in those days – real good neighbours. I mean they'd never let anyone starve. We never used to lock our front doors – not a bit of string or nothing, the house was open day and night ... There were real criminals of course – but never against their own.
>
> (White 1988: 26)

Community life was not always remembered so fondly. Dennis and Daniels report that 'close propinquity, together with cultural poverty, led as much to enmity as it did to friendship'.[1] They assert that communities 'may be characterised as much by antagonism, jealousy, fear, and suspicion as by more neighbourly attitudes and relationships' (1996: 222). Bornat (1997) agrees. She points out that lack of privacy and physical space meant that community could be an oppressive experience, especially from the perspective of its more junior members who had less power and control over their lives. Community also brought with it discrimination and exclusion for some people, as demonstrated in the growing numbers of accounts of the experiences of minority ethnic groups in Britain. Bornat observes that in the memory of white working-class people, issues of 'race' and ethnicity are in the main absent. In contrast, the experience of members of minority ethnic groups was framed by 'the constraining force of an opposing community whose identity is delineated as other' (1997: 27). It is not only minority ethnic accounts that have been largely missing from community history: the voices of disabled children and adults, and stories of gay and lesbian life have also only emerged in recent years (1997: 28).

Traditional sociological approaches

Functionalist approaches

Functionalist perspectives, as we will see, stress the importance of community for the well-being of society as a whole. It is argued that industrialisation and urbanisation damaged the ties that bind communities together, and that new ways needed to be found to help communities to regain their former sense of shared identity and collaborative concern.

Gemeinschaft and Gesellschaft

The nineteenth-century German sociologist Ferdinand Tonnies has had an enduring influence on sociological and everyday ideas about community, past and present. Writing in *Gemeinschaft and Gesellschaft*, first published in 1877, Tonnies set out to make sense of the changes that he saw taking place in Europe as it was developing from a pre-industrial to an industrial society. Tonnies conceptualised the changes primarily as changes in social relationships, from 'Gemeinschaft' to 'Gesellschaft' (roughly translated as 'community' and 'association'). He argued that the quality and nature of social relationships were being transformed by industrialisation, from small-scale, personal, intimate and enduring 'gemeinschaftlich' relationships to individualistic, large-scale, impersonal, calculative and contractual 'gesellschaftlich' relationships. He writes:

> All intimate, private and exclusive living together ... is ... life is Gemeinschaft. Gesellschaft is public life – it is the world itself. In Gemeinschaft with one's family, one lives from birth on, bound to it in weal and woe. One goes into Gesellschaft as one goes into a strange country ... Gemeinschaft is old; Gesellschaft is new ... all praise of rural life has pointed out that the Gemeinschaft among

people is stronger there and more alive; it is the lasting and genuine form of living together. In contrast to Gemeinschaft, Gesellschaft is transitory and superficial. Accordingly, Gemeinschaft should be understood as a living organism, Gesellschaft as a mechanical aggregate and artefact.

(1955: 37–9)

The quotation makes it abundantly clear that Tonnies regretted what he saw as the passing of Gemeinschaftlich relationships. In Gemeinschaft, people knew who they were; they knew their place in life; beliefs and values were clear and well-internalised; and there was a strong value placed on kinship, territory, and solidarity. Industrialisation was changing all this, Tonnies believed, and was bringing about the decline of community in the modern world. Significantly, Tonnies asserts that there are elements of Gemeinschaft and Gesellschaft in all social relationships and in all societies; they should not be understood as exclusive categories, but rather as tendencies or influences that pervade different societies in varying degrees. But he also admits that he saw a greater tendency towards Gemeinschaft in rural areas. This has led some sociologists, as we shall see, to equate Gemeinschaft with the countryside and Gesellschaft with the city – the city becomes the symbol of the breakdown of community in the modern world.

Tonnies' work can be compared with Durkheim's classic essay, 'The Division of Labour in Society', first published in 1893, in which he distinguishes between the 'mechanical' solidarity of pre-industrial societies (that is, societies characterised by likeness and shared morality) and the 'organic' solidarity typical of industrial society (with its complex division of labour, specialisation and difference between people). Durkheim argued, like Tonnies, that modern industrial society was becoming more diverse and more complex, and that the changes were leading to individual unhappiness and social disorganisation. (This issue is discussed further in Chapter 7.)

Community as locality: urban studies

The first person to relate the ideas of Gemeinschaft and Gesellschaft to specific localities was Georg Simmel (1858–1917), a German contemporary of Tonnies. Writing in 1903, Simmel characterised urban life as a constantly changing series of encounters (Simmel 1971); this 'rapid crowding of changing images' encouraged people to deal with social situations at a rational, 'head' level, rather than at a more intuitive, or habitual 'heart' level. At the same time, because the city was the centre of the money economy, social relationships were becoming impersonalised and standardised, untouched by the complications and involvement that personal relationships bring. The modern, urban mind was, for Simmel, more calculating; the world a mere arithmetical problem to be solved. Simmel concludes that people were becoming 'blasé' in outlook, reserved and estranged from one another, frantically searching for self-identity and individuality. (There are strong connections here with Durkheim's notion of 'anomie', see pp.171–3.)

Simmel's approach to urbanism was picked up and developed by Louis Wirth, who worked at the University of Chicago's School of Sociology (see Chapter 7 for a fuller discussion of the work of the Chicago School). Wirth believed that urbanisation had had more impact on society than either industrialisation or capitalism, changing social relationships for ever, and displacing human beings from their 'natural' state: 'Nowhere has mankind been further removed from organic nature than under the conditions of life characteristic of great cities ... [the city] wipes out completely the previously dominant modes of human association' (1938: 1–3). Wirth presents the city and the countryside as two opposite poles: when we leave the countryside, we leave not only the physical environment of the countryside but a rural way of life, taking on instead the values and behaviour of urbanism as a way of life. Urbanism is thus a cultural, rather than a physical phenomenon. It controls all economic, political and cultural life, drawing 'even the most remote parts of the world into its orbit' (1938: 2).

Wirth identifies the defining characteristics of the city as:

1   The large size of its population – the increased population results in a high division of labour – people perform specialised roles. As a consequence, we cannot know each other as whole, rounded individuals; our relationships tend to be segmental and 'secondary', related to a person's role such as shop assistant, employer, etc. We have many of these superficial contacts with people and we protect ourselves from the needs and claims of others by appearing reserved or indifferent to them. Urbanism is summed up by Wirth in two different scenarios – first, the experience of loneliness in a crowd, and second, the relationship between the taxi-driver and his fare – a 'brief encounter' which demonstrates all these features.

2   Its high population density – the increased concentration of people in a limited space leads to a range of environmental and sociological problems. Overcrowding and pollution are accompanied by

a rise in social and interpersonal conflict in the ghettos, as well as a greater awareness of the gap between rich and poor in society.

3 Its social diversity – the more diverse and specialised population may allow for more personal freedom and greater choice; it may also contribute to a sense of insecurity and instability. According to Wirth, people living in cities are more likely than those in rural areas to suffer from mental breakdowns, commit suicide or become victims of crime. The individual feels powerless to do anything to improve the patterns of urban life, and so joins groups of like-minded people in an attempt to recreate some sense of order and control.

Community as locality: rural studies

While Wirth was investigating the defining characteristics of urban life in Chicago in the 1920s and 1930s, an anthropologist called Robert Redfield was studying rural communities in Mexico, seeking to identify the qualities of rural life. Redfield described the way of life here as 'folk society':

> Such a society is small, isolated, non-literate and homogeneous, with a strong sense of group solidarity ... Behaviour is traditional, spontaneous, uncritical and personal: there is no legislation or habit of experiment and reflection for intellectual ends. Kinship, its relations and institutions, are the type categories of experience and the familial group is the unit of action.
>
> (1947: 293)

Redfield's 'folk society' has strong connections with Tonnies' concept of Gemeinschaft. It is also very closely related to Wirth's belief that where we live has a profound impact on how we live: that locality determines lifestyle.

Interpretive studies – challenges to the urban/rural polarity

Interpretive studies take as their starting-point the meaning of community, seeking to discover what living in the city and the countryside actually means to people themselves. Gans (1980) rejects Wirth's notion of a distinctively urban way of life, arguing that different ways of life can be distinguished in the city. He points out that the majority of the American city population lived in quite stable, secure communities which protected them from the worst consequences of urban living (Fulcher and Scott 1999: 404). Even those who lived in the inner city were a mixed population, some of whom lived there by choice. Gans discerns five different groups living in the inner city (1968, reprinted in Bocock *et al.* 1980: 400–2):

- The 'cosmopolites': students, writers, artists, intellectuals who live in the inner city to be close to educational and cultural facilities. Many are unmarried or childless. They have no wish to be integrated and have no connections with the neighbourhood in which they live.

- The unmarried or childless: Gans distinguishes two groups here – those who are temporarily childless and living in the inner city and those who will permanently live there. They are geographically mobile workers who again have no interest in their local neighbourhood, and do not suffer from social isolation. (We might call them 'yuppies' today, living in gentrified flats in run-down parts of inner cities.)

- The 'ethnic villagers': groups from a common ethnic background, living in a neighbourhood with strong family and kinship ties, but with little involvement in secondary relationships in the neighbourhood. They are suspicious of others outside their group.

- The 'deprived': 'the very poor, emotionally disturbed or otherwise handicapped', single parent families, and those experiencing racial discrimination, living in the cheapest housing and suffering from social isolation.

- The 'trapped' and downward mobile: those who have no choice about where they live – they stay 'when a neighbourhood is invaded by non-residential land uses or lower status immigrants' or are old people on low incomes who have lost their social ties and experience social isolation.

This is a very different picture to Wirth's pessimistic presentation of urban life. Gans asserts that ways of life have more to do with social class and family cycle stage than with urban or rural location; that there is no such thing as an urban way of life. He observes that some people are protected from the social consequences of living in a city by social class – the higher the income, the greater degree of choice people have over where they live. In addition, stage in the family cycle determines the area of choice within a social class, so that families with young children may only be able to afford to buy a new house on a modern estate. Any similarities between people living in the same area are not, he argues, to do with locality, but are instead the outcome of a series of constrained choices.

As urban studies have come under sustained criticism, so studies of village life have been attacked for their romantic portrayal of a rural idyll. Bell and Newby (1971) discuss the work of anthropologist Oscar Lewis (1949), who published a very different account of life in a Mexican village. Studying the same village (Tepotzlan) as Redfield, Lewis came up with very different results, finding individualism, lack of co-operation, tension, schisms, fear, envy and distrust amongst the inhabitants. Later studies of village life have stressed that there is a high degree of fluidity in relationships in country areas; that they were not necessarily as stable as presented. Others draw attention to the contractual employer–employee nature of rural relationships, which were much more characteristic of Gesellschaft than Gemeinschaft concepts.

Two additional kinds of studies have exploded some of the myths and polarities inherent in urban and rural sociology. Studies of postwar working-class communities have discovered that industrialisation and urbanisation did not bring about a decline in community life as envisaged by the nineteenth-century theorists and their followers (Fulcher and Scott 1999: 415). Instead, features of working-class life actively encouraged the growth of strong communities: workers lived and worked in one area, often for one employer; trade unions encouraged social solidarity, as did the need to rely on one another for support in times of deprivation (1999: 415). Once established, these communities were self-sustaining and able, to a degree, to resist external changes. (See Young and Willmott's 1957 study of Bethnal Green in the East End of London. The authors expected to find evidence that postwar changes had led to a breakdown of community, but instead discovered that Bethnal Green was surprisingly homogeneous and stable, with strong kinship patterns still very much in evidence.)

The growth of the suburbs has also been of great interest to sociologists. There have been many studies of suburbs, some emphasising their homogeneous nature, others their heterogeneity. These studies have pointed out the falsity of the Gemeinschaft/Gesellschaft dichotomy or even seeing it as a continuum. Instead, they argue that both types of relationship can be found in one locality. In addition, the studies have demonstrated that social relationships do not need to be located in one geographical place in order to survive. Bell's (1968) research into a middle-class housing estate in Swansea demonstrates that kinship ties and social networks can be maintained over long distances. Bulmer suggests that this is no longer just a middle-class phenomenon. Increasingly, working-class people live at some distance from their extended family and may only see their relatives at week-

Implications for practice

Community care policies resonate with nostalgic historical and sociological ideas of community: community as a rural Gemeinschaft and community as a tight-knit, postwar working-class neighbour-hood. Bulmer argues that this creates a major problem for practice because the notions and the worlds on which the policies are built simply do not exist in the late twentieth century, if they ever did. Community care social workers must be aware that we cannot rely on either the existence or the continuing survival of reciprocal, supportive relationships between family and neighbours. People's social networks are today more widely spread geographically and at the same time more privatised in the nuclear family. Hence an attempt to foster local attachment is not in any way 'natural': it is not about drawing out attachment which is already there waiting to be used, but Bulmer argues, must be created through new mediating structures (1987: 70).[2]

ends; meanwhile friendship groups become more important on a day-to-day basis (1987: 55).

Critical developments

There have been growing criticisms of the idea that *where* people live determines *how* they live, that locality determines lifestyle, and criticisms too of the romanticism implicit in the earlier studies. Did pre-industrial, feudal society represent a place of contentment and 'communion' with others? Or was it, rather, a society characterised by a struggle for subsistence, in which individuals were tied to their locality by economic interdependence and by legal constraints which forbade them to leave? The 'social lived reality' (Symonds 1998) of community was in practice the total powerlessness of large numbers of people.

There has been criticism too of the representation of working-class communities. What did the closeness and sharing actually mean to those living in, for example, Bethnal Green? Was it really so cosy to have to share washing facilities and toilets? And was the caring community something which everyone participated equally in, or was it rather, largely care by kin, and in this case, women in the family? Again, the 'social lived reality' may have been poverty, lack of transport and lack of alternative housing, not community spirit (Allan 1991: 110).

An alternative approach argues that the community is not about the city, or about the rural–urban dichotomy, or about locality and where we live, or even about social networks as such. Instead it is about wider structural issues such as class, 'race', gender, age, disability. If we are working-class and poor, or old, sick and disabled, or children or women with young children, our community is likely to be restricted to our locality. And because many others in the locality are not oriented to the community in the same way, the traditional support or mutual aid which may have been available in the past cannot be drawn on to the same extent. If we are middle-class, working-class in work, young, mobile, car-owning, our community will be much wider. Jordan (1996) makes the distinction between 'communities of choice' (among mainstream households) and 'communities of fate' (among the poor and excluded). He argues that this polarisation has high social costs, not least in social problems associated with concentrations of deprivation and the expenditure on social control considered necessary to counter these problems (1996: 188).

Class and community

One of the best-known studies of class and community is Rex and Moore's (1967) study of Sparkbrook, a district on the south-east side of Birmingham. Rex and Moore chart the distribution of housing use within Sparkbrook, describing the various movements in and out of the district from the 1930s onwards, as well as describing the area's inhabitants themselves. They notice that different types of housing are used by different groups of people. For example, the large houses in the 'zone of transition',[3] vacated by the middle-classes on their progress out to the more desirable suburbs, had been turned into lodging-houses and occupied by incoming immigrants: first Irish, then European and increasingly in the early 1960s, 'coloured' (sic) immigrants. Rex and Moore distinguish six different housing situations, also referred to as 'housing classes' (1967: 274):

1   that of the outright owner-occupier of a whole house;
2   that of the owner of a mortgaged whole house;

3   that of the council tenant: (a) in a house with a long life; (b) in a
    house awaiting demolition;
4   that of the tenant of a whole house owned by a private landlord;
5   that of the owner of a house bought with short-term loans who is
    compelled to let rooms in order to meet his repayment obliga-
    tions;
6   that of the tenant of rooms in a lodging-house.

Rex and Moore make an important observation. Not only do different
groups of people inhabit different types of housing, this demarcation is
not accidental. It is caused, in part, by local authority housing policies.
Criteria such as the residence rule (which stated that applicants for
council housing must have lived in the area for five years) effectively
excluded minority ethnic people from council housing. This 'left them
to the mercy of the free market' (1967: 260), forcing them into
lodging houses and poor quality accommodation in run-down areas.
Rex and Moore assert that the consequences are damaging for race relations and for the city itself (1967: 265). Rex and Moore's study is
significant in that it makes it clear that structured inequality determines an individual's housing and neighbourhood, not personal choice
or lifestyle. Their work has been criticised, however, for being too
geographically and historically specific, and for misunderstanding
some of the issues for black people, most crucially that Indian and
Pakistani immigrants actually chose to buy larger property in the city
centre because it suited their requirements, rather than because they
were passive victims of housing policy.
    Marxist writers develop the structural analysis, arguing that
lifestyle and community must be explained in terms of class and
factors relating to class in a capitalist society. Harvey writes:
'Urbanism has to be regarded as a set of social relationships which
reflect relationships established throughout society as a whole. Further,
these relationships have to express the laws whereby urban phenomena
are structured, regulated and constructed' (1973: 304). Because of this,
problems such as poverty, housing and crime are not urban problems at
all; they are societal problems revealed in an urban context, their
causes related to capitalism and social and economic inequalities rather
than to urbanisation. Giddens (1982) agrees, asserting that capitalism
has transformed both urban and rural life; that it is wage labour, not
where people live, that shapes their lives.
    Sennett (1977) picks up this theme. He argues importantly that
people have been diverted from the realities of power by an emphasis
on community. He is concerned that, by always looking inward, and

by placing all our faith on our personal, intimate relationships in the family (what he calls 'destructive gemeinschaft'[4]), we fail to give attention to the large-scale forces in society. He expresses this powerfully:

> Localism and local autonomy are becoming widespread political creeds, as though the experience of power relations will have more human meaning the more intimate the scale – even though the actual structures of power grow ever more into an international system. Community becomes a weapon against society, whose great vice is now seen to be its impersonality. But a community of power can only be an illusion in a society like that of the industrial West, one in which stability has been achieved by the progressive extension of the international scale of structures of economic control. In sum, the belief in direct human relations on an intimate scale has seduced us from converting our understanding of the realities of power into guides for our own political behaviour. The result is that the forces of domination or inequity remain unchallenged.
>
> (1977: 339)

'Race'/ethnicity and community

Fulcher and Scott (1999: 430) assert that ethnicity as well as class has provided a basis for city communities. As already mentioned, Gans as early as 1968 had written about ethnic villages with a distinctive way of life based on strongly integrated communities. Rex and Moore (1967) had also explored different ethnic populations living in the 'zone of transition'. Fulcher and Scott suggest that various aspects of the situation of ethnic minorities facilitate community formation: they tend to be geographically concentrated in one area; they have distinctive cultural, linguistic and religious traditions that bind them together; and, crucially, racism plays a key role in determining collective identity. They write:

> Ethnic communities are not just the product of shared customs and beliefs. They are also the result of common experiences of exclusion and discrimination, and the creation of organizations for mutual support and protection.
>
> (1999: 430)

It is not only black communities for whom ethnic identity and ethnicity has provided a sense of community. Fulcher and Scott describe the emergence of 'defended communities' amongst white people in the East End of London and in the Beaumont Leys estate in Leicester, as a result of competition for local jobs and housing. Foster (1996) tells the story of the Isle of Dogs in London's Docklands, where the white working-class residents united against the predominantly Bengali population who had been forced to move into the area because of changes in local authority housing allocation. Foster records that her sympathies initially lay with the indigenous population, but that she had changed her mind: 'The positive sense of "belonging", community and traditional attachment to a way of life valued by some of the indigenous residents had to be weighed against the negativity of a culture which by definition stigmatised, marginalised and was hostile to those who did not "belong" ' (1996: 151).

Fulcher and Scott suggest that recent attempts to reduce ethnic and racial conflict have been successful by fostering interdependence between groups, through an organised initiative such as a sporting activity or improvements in a housing estate (1999: 431). What these initiatives have sought to do is to establish communities on a residential rather than an ethnic basis – taking us directly back to the idea of community as locality.

Gender and community

In investigating community, sociologists and geographers have identified that men and women have very different understandings and experiences of community, in terms of location, social relationships and a sense of identity. While other factors such as class, age, 'race' and ethnicity, and disability inevitably have an impact on men's mobility and resources, men's communities have nevertheless been found to be much broader and more diverse than those of women. Men are more likely to work and live in different areas, and may choose to socialise and take part in leisure and sport activities across community boundaries. Women are more likely to make more use of their local communities, as Cornwell's (1984) study in East London demonstrates. Women here occupied a much wider range of communal spaces than men – 'the shops, the street, the school gates, their relatives' houses' – and they had a much wider variety of contacts, 'not only with shopkeepers and other mothers, but also in the schools, pubs and blocks of flats where many of them are employed as cleaners' (1984: 50).

Williams (1997) considers how far women's centredness in their locality actually represents an exclusion from the outside world. She points out that factors such as poverty, lack of time and independent transport, the identification of leisure facilities as men's spaces (pubs, clubs and playing fields) and fear of violence or racial or sexual assault can confine women to their local neighbourhoods. Yet women have also been able to turn this confinement to their own ends, developing supportive relationships or getting involved in community action to fight for safer roads, for nursery provision, etc. Williams suggests that community has particular significance for many women: 'It is the point of negotiation over public provision; it is a site of organisation and struggle over welfare issues; and it is the arena of paid, unpaid and low-paid work' (1997: 34). It marks the overlap for women between private and public issues, between the personal and the political. Women as a result have a contradictory relationship with community: community as the 'space that women struggle to define as theirs', and community as the 'place to which women are confined' (1997: 42–3).

Evans and Fraser (1996) are also interested in the gendered nature of communities, this time focusing on the use of public space in two English cities, Manchester and Sheffield. They highlight four very different popu-lations who make use of the town centres, shopping malls and major thoroughfares in these cities during the daytime and in the evenings: youth, gay men, shoppers and women. Of the four groups, only two (youth and gay men) have been able to develop their own spaces within the public arena, creating their own safe areas. For example, a gay village has developed in Manchester, with its own gay bars, clubs and shops: 'rather than being seen as a "gay ghetto", it is seen as a gay developed space, a place of ownership, a place of which to be proud' (1996: 117). Although used by some lesbian women, this area has developed mainly as a space for gay men. The other two groups (shoppers and women) have not been able to create their own spaces in the same way. The shoppers are split between those who can afford to shop at the up-market, American-style malls and those who are forced to use the declining city centres. Women's use of public space varies considerably according to the time of day. While almost half of those using the public spaces during the daytime are women, they constitute less than one-third of those using these areas in the evenings.

What Evans and Fraser's research demonstrates is the continuing control and dominance of men on public spaces in cities. Campbell (1993) also highlights the importance of gender differences in an anal-ysis of community in her account of the riots in the early 1990s in the working-class housing estates on the outskirts of Newcastle, Oxford and Cardiff. She writes:

The angry young men victimised the women, the neighbours, the community ... The unruly women ... had babies, made relationships, put food on the table, they had cooperated and organised and created community politics.

(1993: 244–5)

Campbell conceptualises the destructiveness and brutality of young men as an attempt to reassert the power and privilege that had been lost along with the 'respectable' working-class neighbourhood, with its community facilities, clubs and employment.

Nation and community

We cannot consider community without giving attention to community in its larger sense: community and nation, or rather, nation as community. Anderson (1991) defines the nation as an 'imagined community': *'imagined* because the members of even the smallest nation will never know most of their fellow-members, meet them, or even hear of them, yet in the minds of each lives the image of their communion' (1991: 6). Anderson argues that all communities larger than primordial villages of face-to-face contact (and perhaps even these) are imagined; what distinguishes one community from another is the style in which they are imagined (ibid.). He continues:

The nation is imagined as *limited* because even the largest of them ... has finite, if elastic, boundaries, beyond which lie other nations ... It is imagined as *sovereign* because the concept was born in an age in which Enlightenment and Revolution were destroying the legitimacy of the divinely-ordained, hierarchical dynastic realm ... nations dream of being free, and, if under God, directly so ... Finally, it is imagined as a *community* because, regardless of the actual inequality and exploitation that may prevail in each, the nation is always conceived as a deep, horizontal comradeship. Ultimately it is this fraternity that makes it possible, over the past two centuries, for so many millions of people, not so much to kill, as willingly to die for such limited imaginings.

(1991: 7)

This, then, is the main focus of Anderson's enquiry: to reflect on why so many people have been willing to make the sacrifice of dying for their 'imagined community'. McCrone's (1992) study of Scotland provides further insight. McCrone calls Scotland a nation without a state, or a 'stateless nation'; it lacks the political and economic control over its own affairs that is normally associated with nationhood. But Scotland as a country, he argues, is more than simply a geographical place. It is 'a landscape of the mind, a place of the imagination' (1992: 17). As Scotland lost its identity politically, culturally and economically, so it appropriated another vision, 'the Gaelic vision', further appropriated and incorporated into the twentieth-century tourist vision of Scotland (1992: 18). McCrone argues that the inventing of traditions and the creation of myths is not peculiar only to Scotland: 'myth-history' is a vital part of the story-telling of any country, and traditions themselves serve a positive function in legitimising institutions, symbolising group cohesion and socialising others into values and beliefs. Similarly, McCrone rejects the idea that nationalism is always reactionary or atavistic (1992: 206). He argues that there is no 'single' explanation of nationalism, nor one single type. Above all, he writes, 'nationalism, or national identity, is not a characteristic, but imputes a relationship between different identities. To be Scottish, for example, is to be not English' (1992: 207). This reminds us of one of the key points in the discussion of community, that is, that community is about creating and maintaining the boundary between 'us' and 'them', as much as about a specific quality or sentiment shared by 'us'. Territory and boundaries are not real in themselves but are socially created and recreated in our encounters with those on the other side of the divide.

Globalisation and community

Fulcher and Scott (1999: 457–8) outline the main forms taken by globalisation as follows:

- Global organisation (seen initially in the context of the overseas empires of nation-states, but today encompassing transnational corporations and international organisations, both of which challenge the nation-state's control of national economies);
- Global interdependence (the growth of the world economy is one of the main aspects of the globalisation process);
- Global communication (telecommunications and information technology allow different parts of the world to be closely connected with one another, so that people, money and information can move rapidly around the world, raising the question of whether states can any longer control their boundaries);

- Global awareness (advances in technology mean that people are now more aware of the world as a whole; they therefore see themselves more as human beings and less as members of this community or that country).

Some sociologists argue that globalisation has led to the decline of the nation-state, with its separate territory, citizens and administration. Others disagree, arguing that global organisations will continue to be dependent on nation-states for their functioning (Fulcher and Scott 1999: 459). It seems likely that both statements may be true: that while the world gets smaller daily, and the power of multi-national

---

Implications for practice

It has been argued that an individual's experience of community is shaped by structural factors such as class, 'race'/ethnicity and gender. The idea of community is itself created by exclusion and separateness as much as by shared identity and culture. This has important implications for practice. In attempting to build community solidarity, we need to be aware of the dangers within this, since it is the perceived differences between 'us' and 'them' that strengthen our sense of 'us'. Communities may be very intolerant of differences between community members, just as they are likely to amplify the differences between those 'inside' and those 'outside' the community. This means that racism, sexism and heterosexism might be as much a part of community identity as togetherness and generosity of spirit.

Patel (1990) argues that community imagery is largely Eurocentric, taking little account of the differing needs of black people, or of the pre-existing supportive and defensive networks operating within ethnic minority groups. It is also largely heterosexist, giving little attention to other supportive arrangements, for example those that exist in the gay community. These ideas will be explored more fully in the next chapter.

---

companies grows, so people will wish to look for meaning in their lives through the very myths and traditions that are the heart of imagined community. This means that in the future, while seeing ourselves as part of a world-wide social network (a 'global village') we may at the same time develop stronger ties with those around us; our sense of shared identity may be consolidated on a more local basis.

Conclusion

I have argued in this chapter that, while it is easy to be in favour of the idea of community, in practice community is a highly problematic concept. Community is as much about social polarisation and exclusion as it is about mutuality and neighbourliness; the flip side of community may be racism, insularity, sexism, coercion, or simply nosiness, lack of privacy, disruption and interference. Whether we understand community as a geographical locality, social network or sense of identity, it has the capacity to be used both positively and negatively. As Jordan writes, 'community can serve to integrate membership groups with antagonistic interests, and to mobilize them for conflict, rather than sustain programmes for harmonization and inclusion' (1996: 164).

Recommended reading

- Bornat, J., Johnson, J., Pereira, C., Pilgrim, D. and Williams, F. (1997) *Community Care: A Reader*, Second edition, Basingstoke: Macmillan, in association with the Open University (this is a collection of readings that covers the whole field of community and caring well).
- Bulmer, M. (1987) *The Social Basis of Community Care*, London: Allen and Unwin (a readable account).
- Patel, N. (1990) *'Race' against Time: Social Services Provision to Black Elders*, London: Runnymede Trust (a good antidote to the Eurocentric literature on community care).

6 Caring

Introduction

The focus of this chapter is a sociological examination of the concept of caring. Unlike other chapters in the book, the period under scrutiny is relatively short, from the mid-1970s to the present day. This is because, up until the mid-1970s, caring was largely unproblematised in sociology, hidden in the family and in normative, functionalist notions about women and women's role in the family and society. The newness of caring as a topic of sociological investigation should not, however, lead the reader to assume that the field of enquiry is a small one. There has been a huge amount of empirical research and sociological theorising about caring over the last twenty years or so. Much of this analysis, particularly in the early stages, has its roots in feminist writing and action. More recently, the debates have been driven by disabled writers and by a wider structural perspective – one which forefronts the importance of 'race', class, age and disability, as well as gender issues.

The chapter makes a deliberate distinction between care (the institutional site where caring takes place) and caring (an act carried out by one person for another, with physical, emotional, social and even spiritual dimensions). While there has been some important sociological examination of care (for example, Goffman 1968 and Townsend 1962), as well as extensive discussion of the professional base of social work (for example, Davies 1991, Dominelli 1997), I have chosen to concentrate in this chapter on caring, rather than care. This is because of the relevance of an exploration of caring for community care practice today across all care settings, whether they are family-based, day-care or residential, paid or unpaid, professional, volunteer or low-paid domestic service.

The emergence of caring as a subject of sociological interest in the mid-1970s both reflects and anticipates wider political, social and economic changes. From the 1960s onwards, feminist sociologists and psychologists had been asking fundamental questions about the relationship between women's private and public lives, seeking to challenge the sexual division of labour in the home and in society. Studies of mothering, housework, and gender socialisation demonstrate the beginnings of this new field of research and analysis (for example, Oakley 1974, Baker Miller 1978, and Chodorow 1978). Just as important, however, was the beginning of a disability rights' movement, a movement which challenged the 'personal tragedy theory of disability' (Oliver 1990) and put in its place a campaign for civil rights for people with disabilities. It was the Union of the Physically Impaired against Segregation, set up in 1974, that first defined disability as being socially caused, and acted to spearhead a collective struggle for change (Davis 1996: 126–7).

Demographic changes also forced the issue of caring onto the academic (and government) agenda. While women's rights and the rights of disabled people were being championed, so forecasts of escalating costs of meeting the health and welfare needs of older people strengthened the UK government's preference for community care (Arber and Ginn 1992b: 86). Henwood (1990) reports that the total population of disabled and older people increased by nearly one-third between 1961 and 1981. Although the overall increase was expected to slow down between 1981 and 2001, the proportion of very elderly people (and hence those most likely to need some form of assistance and care) was expected to more than double. As older people were living longer (and, it was suggested, living longer with increasing ill-health), so divorce and women's employment outside the home were increasing, raising fears about how care needs might be met in the future. In consequence, we can identify a qualitative shift in the meaning of community care during the 1970s, from care 'in' the community to care 'by' the community (this theme is pursued later in the chapter; see pp.163–5).

There is not space in this chapter to review the whole field of sociological research and literature on caring. I will, however, identify and discuss the key debates around the concept of caring. I will examine the literature in terms of two distinct phases of sociological enquiry: first, studies from the 1980s which owe allegiance to a feminist framework of analysis and focus largely on carers' experiences; and second, studies from the 1990s which criticise the early analysis for what is perceived to be a very 'one-sided account of the caring relationship' (Arber and Ginn 1992b: 87).

The development of a feminist critique of caring

Three interrelated questions are addressed in the early sociological literature on caring: Who cares? What is caring? Why do people (understood largely as women) care?

Who cares?

The starting-point for the problematisation of caring lies in an Equal Opportunities Commission (EOC) research study and a polemic article by Finch and Groves, both published in 1980, and both drawing attention to the fact that caring is something which is done mainly by women. The EOC study was based on a postal questionnaire to 2,500 randomly selected households in West Yorkshire. The study found that, of the 116 people identified as carers, 75 per cent were women and 25 per cent men. An EOC report, published two years later, estimated from this that there were 1.25 million female carers in Britain.[1] Soon afterwards, a Women and Employment Survey (1984) found that 13 per cent of all women had caring responsibilities for sick or elderly dependants (Martin and Roberts 1984).[2]

Finch and Groves' (1980) article set the parameters of the feminist critique of caring. They are highly scathing about the discrepancy between a government commitment to equal opportunities for women and men (as evidenced by legislation) and community care policies that rely on women's unpaid domestic labour. They argue that the two cannot go together: policies for community care were, within a context of public expenditure cuts, incompatible with policies for equal opportunities for women. They summarise with what has become a much quoted equation: 'that in practice, community care equals care by the family, and in practice care by the family equals care by women' (1980: 494).

Other feminist writers have taken up the issue of caring in different ways. Wilson (1982) asserts that older people are not being cared for by the 'community': 'They are being cared for exclusively and predominantly by their daughters and daughters-in-law.' She urges that the term 'community' be abandoned altogether as a 'veil of illusion' which cocoons and oppresses women (1982: 55). Finch, even more contentiously, proposes that, in order to safeguard the position of women, residential and institutional care should be extended as an alternative to community care. She argues that there can be no non-sexist version of community care; informal care inevitably falls on women and women's networks. Because of this, 'the residential route is the only one which ultimately will offer us a way out of the impasse of caring' (1984: 16). Dalley (1988) agrees with this position. She asserts that social policy must develop along collectivist principles, in place of the familist and individualist principles that motivate community care policies.

A number of qualitative studies of women carers affirm the feminist position on caring, including Brody (1981) on 'women in the middle', caught at a time in their lives between caring for children and parents at the same time; Lewis and Meredith (1988) on daughters who care; Glendinning (1992) on the costs of care-giving; and Nissel and Bonnerjea (1982) on caring for older relatives.

What is caring?

An important issue for the unfolding sociological analysis of caring has been the exploration of the nature of caring itself, that is, what is caring? Sociologists have drawn attention to the fact that caring is work, although often unseen and unrecognised as such. This subject was first exposed in Oakley's (1974) investigation of housework. It was then developed by Roy Parker (1981) in terms of caring for an older person. Parker makes the distinction between caring for and caring about someone: while friendship typically involves the former, it does not usually involve the latter. Caring for someone, he suggests, 'comprises such things as feeding, washing, lifting, protecting, representing and comforting' (1981: 3). All these tasks take time, and the time cannot be used for anything else. Caring about someone, in contrast, does not use up time in this way. Thus caring for someone, he argues, should be re-named 'tending' a person, since it is a time-consuming activity that takes place in the context of obligations that are socially, not affectively, constructed. The idea of caring as 'tending' has been taken up by feminist writers including Ungerson (1983).

Graham takes issue with Parker's conceptualisation. For Graham, caring is more than 'a kind of domestic labour performed on people ... Caring cannot be understood objectively and abstractly, but only as a subjective experience in which we are all, for better or worse involved' (1983: 27–8). Drawing on the analyses of Baker Miller (1978) and Chodorow (1978), Graham considers the ways in which caring is a fundamental part of female self-identity. The caring role, she advises, is reproduced in women themselves through the dynamics of the mother–daughter relationship. It is also linked to the wider sexual division of labour in society:

[It is] constructed through a network of social and economic relations, both within the home and the workplace, in which women
take responsibility for meeting the emotional and material needs
not only of husbands and children, but of the elderly, the handicapped, the sick and the unhappy.

(1983: 22)

Graham argues for a reconception of caring, one that takes on board
'both love and labour, both identity and activity' (1983: 13). Caring,
she suggests, is a work-role 'whose form and content is shaped (and
continually re-shaped) by our intimate, social and sexual relationships'
(1983: 29). It is also the medium through which women gain access to
both the private and the public world, as wives and mothers, secre-
taries and social workers. She concludes:

caring defines both the identity and the activity of women in
Western society. It defines what it feels like to be a woman in a
male-dominated and capitalist social order ... Thus, caring is not
something on the periphery of our social order; it marks the point
at which the relations of capital and gender intersect.

(1983: 30)

Graham's article has proved to be extremely influential and also
controversial, for feminists and sociologists alike. Conflict between the
idea of caring as work and caring as identity has remained a live issue
in the caring literature. Graham has herself shifted her position considerably in recent years, as we will discuss later.

Why do people care?

Feminist and other sociological studies conducted in the 1980s offer a
range of explanations for why people care, many of them overlapping
with each other, and with gender-based analyses to the fore.

Practical considerations

Some research has focused on the impact of practical exigencies in
determining whether or not people care for others. For example,
studies have considered the number of people in the household ('is
there space for granny?'), geographical proximity (is daily or weekly
care feasible and possible?). Research has shown that physical proximity is not the only reason for caring. Abrams (1978; Abrams *et al.*

1989) in a study of neighbourhood care found that, although living near someone may facilitate the giving of help, it does not determine that help will be given in the first place. They argue that informal neighbourhood caring is activated primarily as a result of an existing social context within which resources, relationships and culture enable or impede help among people because they are neighbours. In addition, physical space (or the lack of it) seems to bear little relation on whether or not care is given.

Time and opportunity

Another way of answering this question might be to think about who in the family has actual time or opportunity to care. Ungerson (1983) demonstrates that this issue is fundamentally connected with women and women's place at home and in the labour market. She argues that women's unequal position in the labour market makes it likely that for a married couple, the most 'rational' decision is usually that the women should give up work to look after a relative in need of care. This in turn reinforces the general belief that caring is women's work. She writes: 'The ideology of housework and women's place within it has a material impact on women's paid work which in turn serves to reinforce that very ideology' (1983: 38).

It might be expected that, with the impact of rising male unemployment, and women's greater participation in the workforce, more men might become involved in caring responsibilities. Findings from research suggests that this may not be the case. Nissel and Bonnerjea's innovative (1982) study used time diaries with forty-four married couple households caring for an older dependent relative. They found that wives spent on average between two and three hours every day undertaking essential care for the relative, irrespective of whether or not they were in paid employment. The husbands, in contrast, spent only eight minutes. This finding is reflected in studies of men and women's involvement in housework in dual income families. Hochschild (1990) observes that it is women who are most likely to do 'the second shift' – preparing the evening meal, loading the washing machine and getting up in the night for a sick child. Interestingly, Qureshi and Walker's study of fifty-eight carers found that working sons were more likely to provide assistance to elderly parents than unemployed sons: nearly two in five did so as compared with only one in five unemployed sons (1989: 115).

By accident

Some people (men and women) find themselves caring for someone by accident. They may have never left home, and find themselves in adulthood caring for an elderly or sick parent. Many others find themselves in a caring role when a partner (or parent) becomes sick or disabled.

Fay Wright's (1986) research into single people caring for relatives found that, whilst women and men both cared for their relatives in this situation, gender played a significant part in determining the kind of care that was sought and given. In her study, mothers living with sons were less dependent than those living with daughters. She also established that caring for a parent affected women's employment far more than men's; they were more likely to go part-time and even give up work completely to care for a relative. Perhaps surprisingly, she discovered that sons received less help from kin and neighbours, because they were less likely to be plugged into informal caring networks and exchanges.

For money

Some people care for others for money. It is the decrease in availability of women to carry out unpaid caring which has forced the government to look at ways of encouraging women back into caring through financial inducements. More women are working, full and part-time;[3] fewer women are at home caring for children and dependent relatives (and so available for volunteering); more women are married (so there are fewer single daughters around); and more women are living too far away to provide daily or even weekly care. The family may not be able to continue to meet its own needs for care, never mind take on caring for others. As a consequence, there has been a steady expansion in new schemes to pay carers, such as community care schemes which pay relatives for expenses only, and schemes in which 'ordinary people' provide live-in and foster-care situations for an increasingly wide range of client groups (Leat and Gay 1987).

Affect and reciprocity

In an early study, Abrams (1978) suggests that affect and reciprocity are important determinants of informal helping; in other words, we care for those we like, and those who we feel a debt of gratitude towards. Qureshi and Walker (1989) surveyed 300 people aged seventy-five or over living in Sheffield in 1982/3 and conducted follow-up interviews with fifty-eight informal carers. They investigated both affect and reciprocity: first, in questions about emotional closeness and shared interests between the older person and their helper, and second, in questions about past and present help given by the older person to the helper. Their findings suggest that neither affect nor reciprocity is essential for the provision of practical care or tending. Although affect and reciprocity are extremely important in determining the nature of the caring experience, they do not determine the actual supply of practical assistance.

Duty and obligation

Duty and obligation are closely linked to the idea of reciprocity, and are rooted in societal and kinship norms. In Qureshi and Walker's (1989) study, both care-givers and care-recipients agreed that caring needs should be met first and foremost in the family. They went on to identify a hierarchy in decision-making about who the carer should be, based firmly on traditional (and Western), normative expectations of kinship obligations. Perhaps surprisingly, gender was not the most important determinant of the obligation to care. Instead, marital relationship and long-term co-residence took precedence over gender. Although the hierarchical principles could be overruled by the ill-health of prospective helpers, they suggest that the following model largely holds true (1989: 126):

1 Spouse (or relative in a lifelong joint household)
2 Daughter
3 Daughter-in-law
4 Son
5 Other relative
6 Non-relative.

Critique of the 1980s studies

Although the 1980s studies have made a significant contribution towards an understanding of the concept and reality of caring, there have nevertheless been a number of fundamental objections to the framework and conclusions of many of the early studies. The objections have centred on three main criticisms. First, it is suggested that by focusing on the experiences of carers and the perceived 'burden' of care, the early studies ignored the perspectives of care-recipients, and the importance of the two-way relationship between carer and recipient.

This has been seriously challenged by sociologists and by disabled people themselves (for example, Fisher 1997, Morris 1991, 1995 and 1997). Second, it is argued that, by concentrating on the kin care provided by women carers (specifically, Brody's 1981 'women in the middle'), the early studies lost sight of other people who care (notably male spouses, sons, children and other older people), as well as the paid carers who work in different settings. In reviewing the early studies, Thomas concludes that the very narrow characterisation of caring led to a 'partial and fragmented understanding of society's caring activity' (1993: 667). Third, it is suggested that, by creating an analytical framework that was premised largely on the accounts of white, middle-aged women, the studies failed to take account of the importance of class, 'race'/ethnicity, gender and sexuality, age, disability and mental health in structuring experiences of caring. Graham (1997) argues that academic feminism has masked issues of 'race' and class, sexuality and disability as crucial mechanisms in women's lives. By concentrating on the experiences of some women (that is, predominantly white, middle-class, care-giving women), feminists have left some women, some relationships and some experiences 'on the margins of analysis' (Graham 1997: 126–7).

New approaches

Recent sociological research into caring challenges much of the received wisdom of the 1980s studies and takes forward the understanding of caring into new areas.

Research on care-recipients

Studies that examine the experiences and feelings of those who are cared for by others paint a very different picture to the one we have already presented. This research demonstrates that many of those who receive care (that is, older people and those with physical disabilities and mental health problems) also continue to care for others in spite of their disabilities, caring for a child, grandchild or older person, preparing meals, doing housework, etc. In consequence, there is a much less clear division between care-giver and care-recipient, or to use more emotive language, between 'carer' and 'dependant'.

This is clearly evidenced by General Household Survey (GHS) statistics.[4] The 1990 GHS suggests that as many as 44 per cent of co-resident carers are over sixty-five years of age; similarly, the OPCS Disability Survey estimates that 40 per cent of main carers for disabled adults are over sixty-five (Clarke 1995: 24). It is also demonstrated by qualitative studies of care-recipients. Morris observes that none of the disabled people whom she interviewed for her study referred to family members who helped them as 'carers'; they talked about their relationships with their partners, children, parents and friends, not their 'carers' (1995: 90). Caring is therefore not a 'one-way street': people care for each other in what is frequently a shared, reciprocal relationship. (This connects strongly with elements in Graham's 1983 analysis.)

Research studies also show that people who may require care hold onto their independence for as long as they can, struggling alone at home, or in the marital relationship, before admitting that they need help. The older people surveyed by Qureshi and Walker (1989) were acutely aware that they did not wish to become a burden to their children. They write: 'Elderly people do not give up their independence easily; with few exceptions they are reluctant subjects in caring and dependency' (1989: 18–19). When care was inevitable, they preferred their care needs to be met in the family, first and foremost by their spouse or an adult who shared their household. Arber and Ginn (1992: 93), drawing on their own earlier research and on wider literature, offer a new hierarchy of older people's preferences for care contexts:

A   In elderly person's own home – self care
B   In elderly person's own home – care provided by co-resident

    (i)   Spouse
    (ii)   Other same-generation relative
    (iii) Child or non-kin.

C   In elderly person's own home – care provided by extra-resident

    (iv)   Child
    (v)   Other relative
    (vi)   Neighbour, friend, volunteer.

D   In care-giver's own home

    (vii) Unmarried child
    (viii) Married child.

This model confirms Qureshi and Walker's broad findings, but provides new insight into the experience of receiving care. Care preferences can be understood as being based largely on a context of care where the older person feels that they can hold onto the freedom and integrity that they enjoyed in the past. Studies of care preferences of people with disabilities shed further light on this issue. This literature suggests that some care-recipients may prefer to receive at least some of their care from a person outside their family, for example, a volunteer or a paid professional (Clarke 1995: 30). This allows them to feel more independence and autonomy, and enables them to protect the balance of their personal relationships. Morris (1995) cites the views of one disabled care-recipient, Catherine:

> It's very difficult to ask somebody that you're also in a loving rela-tionship with, it's very difficult to constantly ask them for the basic things you need. I find it's a sort of breath of fresh air in a way when my helper comes in and I have loads and loads of different things that I couldn't ask Robert to do ... I know that there'll be no strings, no other strings attached to the asking, it's just a straight can you do that.
>
> (1995: 86)

This quotation clearly refutes the notion that unpaid 'family' care is always somehow superior to professional or paid care. It also resonates with Parker's (1981) conceptualisation of caring as 'work'.

The 'burden' of caring?

Fisher (1994) asserts that the idea that caring is a 'burden' has a long history in British social policy. He criticises this for three main reasons. First, many carers, both men and women, feel that they have 'chosen' their role; 'they would not have it any other way' (1994: 668). They do not see themselves as passive victims of normative expecta-tions, but have made a positive choice to care. Second, studies demonstrate that caring may be a rewarding experience for carers, when it takes place in the context of an enduring and mutually satis-fying relationship. Third, there is no absolute 'burden' experienced by all. Instead, there are moments when the caring burden seems greatest, at different stages in the caring relationship, and in different ways with different people. Lewis and Meredith (1988) in their study of daugh-ters who care suggest that caring is best understood as a sequence, not a fixed entity, so that a person's need for care is likely to move along a continuum from needing a little care to needing a lot. Likewise, a carer's need for support will change. They urge that care professionals take this into account in making assessments, instead of waiting for support systems to break down before intervening.

Jill Pitkeathly (then Director of the Carers' National Association), interviewed in 1994, agrees. She indicates that it is not the amount of hours put in that is critical, but rather, how the individual carer feels about the caring in which they are involved. From this perspective, an individual who gives a small amount of care might find this more demanding than someone who spends a substantial amount of time in caring. Put simply, experiences of caring inevitably vary (*Community Care*, 10 February 1994: 3).

Obligations reconsidered

Finch and Mason's study of family obligations carried out between 1985 and 1989 explores further the idea of obligations and adult kin relationships. Finch and Mason (1993) studied 978 adults of all ages living in Greater Manchester, seeking to answer three key questions:

1   Do people acknowledge that parent–child relations are founded upon norms of obligation?
2   What is the substance of these norms?
3   How do norms operate in practice?

Finch and Mason found that, at the most general level, most people did assent to the idea of filial obligations, but that this assent was by no means either universal or unconditional. Although there was broad agreement that an adult should 'do something' to support their parents, there was less broad agreement about what exactly that 'something' should be. In reality, people expected to negotiate their obligations; to work out their own responsibilities in a given set of circumstances. Finch and Mason conclude that there may be different ways of fulfilling obligations legitimately: 'People do have an understanding of what would be generally accepted as proper, but they use it as a resource with which to negotiate rather than as a rule to follow' (1993: 105).

Finch (1995) extends this analysis. She suggests that there are different, at times competing expectations of British family life. The idea that 'adult children should be able to live lives independently of their parents and vice-versa' may be just as strong as the notion that children should look after their parents when they become ill or frail. Responsibilities are therefore likely to be tempered on both sides with the desire to retain mutual independence (1995: 51). She proposes an alternative 'commitments' model as a better way of understanding how family responsibilities operate in practice: commitments are built up over time between specific individuals, through contact, shared activities and giving help when it is needed. She states that the process of reciprocity 'is the engine which drives the process of developing commitments' (1995: 54). She ends by suggesting that the idea of fixed obligations may fit spouses better: there may be little room for a spouse to decline to offer care (1995: 54).

Studies of other carers

The notion that it is only women who care has been contested by findings from localised, qualitative studies (for example, Qureshi and Walker 1989, Russell 1983, Wright 1986), and by results and subsequent analysis of information from the UK-wide, quantitative General Household Survey (GHS) (see Arber and Gilbert 1989, Arber and Ginn 1991, Evandrou 1990, Green 1988, Parker 1990, Parker and Lawton 1994).

The 1985 GHS survey showed that one adult in seven in Britain was providing informal care, amounting to 6 million carers overall, with 1.7 million people caring for someone in the same household and 1.4 million spending at least twenty hours per week providing care and support. Of these 6 million carers, 3.5 million were women and 2.5 million were men, although in situations where both husbands and wives were involved in caring, women were more likely to carry main responsibility for caring. Two-thirds of carers were looking after someone who was elderly; the rest were physically and mentally disabled adults and children, the mentally ill, and those with chronic disease or terminal illness. Whilst individuals aged forty-five to fifty-nine years were most likely to have caring responsibilities, 42 per cent of all carers were over retirement age. The majority of caring was directed at relatives, particularly parents or parents-in-law (46 per cent), although nearly 20 per cent of carers cared for a friend. Carers caring for someone in the same household were mainly caring for spouses (40 per cent), for parents (23 per cent) or for children (19 per cent).

Latest figures from the 1990 data suggest an even higher overall number of carers: 6.8 million carers of whom 3.9 million are women and 2.9 million men (Clarke 1995: 20).[5] Figures suggest that there has been a significant rise in the proportion of people who care for an elderly person who does not live with them: the proportion of co-resident carers decreased from 20 per cent in 1985 to 17 per cent in 1990. Most care for older people who are not co-resident: 83 per cent in 1990. Caring for an older person who is co-resident is far more time-consuming than caring for someone who is not: an average of 53 hours a week is spent in caring for a person who is co-resident as compared with 9 hours caring per week for someone living elsewhere. Whilst women provide the largest amounts of care at the forty-five to sixty-four years age-group, elderly men provide more care than middle-aged men. A third of care is provided by older people themselves, mainly spouses, and about half of these are men. Men are more likely to be co-resident carers, either because they are single and have never left home or because they are caring for an elderly spouse.

The results of the GHS studies have proved controversial amongst carers' organisations, social policy analysts and sociologists alike. The issue of gender in caring will be explored later in the chapter. However, it is important at this point to state that a major area of dispute has been about the lack of differentiation between the scale and nature of various care-giving tasks in counting the total numbers of carers. It is argued, for example, that the GHS should differentiate between someone who is doing a little gardening or light shopping and someone who is changing soiled sheets – these are qualitatively different kinds of caring. Parker and Lawton (1994) see this in terms of a distinction between personal and physical care and between 'caring' and 'informal helping'. They estimate that there are only 1.7 million carers heavily involved in 'hands-on' care. Over and above this, there are gender differences here: women are more likely to provide both personal and physical care, whereas men are more likely to provide physical care and/or practical help and less likely to provide personal care.

In recent years there has also been recognition that a substantial amount of caring is carried out by children and young people, most often caring for a disabled or ill parent who lives with them. New research studies have begun to explore the impact caring has on the lives of children and young people, often referred to as 'young carers' (Aldridge and Becker 1993 and 1996, Becker, Aldridge and Deardon 1998, Heron 1998). This research has itself proved controversial, because it has been seen to focus again on the 'burden' of care and the detrimental impact caring has on children, instead of viewing the caring relationship as a complex and reciprocal one (Morris 1997, Olsen 1996).

Structural constraints on caring

Social class

Studies suggest that interrelated factors such as class, income, health and housing play a key part in determining experiences of care and caring. Importantly, while working-class people are likely to have fewer resources and poorer health than middle-class people, research demonstrates that it is working-class families who are more likely to take in an older relative who needs care. It is suggested that this reflects both the lack of viable alternatives (in terms of paying for care) as well as specific ideas about family responsibilities and about the value of independence (Arber and Ginn 1992a). There are age differences here too, in that working-class people are more likely to need care at an earlier age than middle-class people, because of inequalities in health, housing, diet, etc.

In addition, informal caring has a significant impact on household income. Parker and Lawton's (1994) analysis of the 1985 GHS indicates that household incomes of people who live with the person they are caring for are substantially lower than similar households in the general population. Caring is itself expensive, and while the person who is cared for may contribute financially to the costs of their care, this may not cover all the necessary extras, such as household adaptations, extra heating, additional laundry, etc. (Glendinning 1992). Parker and Lawton conclude that the impact of caring on the income and savings of carers may be such that this has serious consequences for their own standard of living in old age.

Research into neighbourhood care suggests that middle-class communities may be more neighbourly than working-class communities (see Abrams *et al.* 1989). There is an important issue here, however. How far does 'neighbourliness' equate with 'caring'? Abrams and his colleagues found that relationships between neighbours are characterised mostly by what they call 'friendly distance': we are happy to water our neighbours' plants while they are on holiday, but less likely to wish to be involved in routine personal care tasks.

If we widen the concept of care to include paid care, and specifically waged domestic labour, issues of class again come to the fore. Graham (1991 and 1997) argues that care cannot be understood without reference to social divisions constructed around 'race' and class as well as gender. Her study of domestic service points out that the burden of low-paid domestic service has always been carried by working-class, often black or immigrant women. In the seventeenth and eighteenth centuries, black slaves were brought to Britain from Africa and the West Indies to work as personal and household servants, as cooks, maids and valets. In the nineteenth century, Afro-Caribbean women continued to be employed as domestic servants in middle-class households, as well as white working-class women and Irish and other minority ethnic groups, who entered domestic service in large numbers. Today domestic service continues to characterise the labour market for many black and white working-class women, engaged in low-paid, low-status jobs in households, in the health and social services and in private care homes (1997: 130).

Gregson and Lowe's (1994) investigation of waged domestic labour (nannies and cleaners) in contemporary Britain adds to this analysis. Gregson and Lowe argue that the resurgence of waged domestic labour in the 1980s and 1990s is indicative of 'a breakdown in the post-war cross-class identification of women with all forms of reproductive work' (1994: 233). As women have entered the paid workforce in greater numbers, so they have relinquished part of their traditional reproductive labour to others, that is, to lower middle-class and working-class women.

Gregson and Lowe assert that a 'class-mediated hierarchy of domestic tasks' is once more being constructed. At the top are the tasks that middle-class partners (women and men) are more or less happy to share, and these tasks remain unwaged, for example, some childcare activities, shopping and cooking. Below this are the routine, day-to-day domestic tasks such as daily childcare and feeding. These are largely shared by middle-class women and waged domestic labour. At the bottom are the labour intensive activities (notably cleaning and ironing) that are increasingly being identified with waged domestic labour from the working-class. The consequence of this is that working-class women, as well as carrying the burden of reproductive work in their own households, are increasingly assuming part of the same responsibility within middle-class households (1994: 234).

This has major implications for our discussion of women and caring. Graham (1997: 130) states that many white working-class women and black and ethnic minority women have found that their care arrangements are structured by employment opportunities and immigration restrictions in ways that restrict their opportunity to receive and give care within their families. It is therefore white middle-class women who have greater access to a family life sustained by their care.

'Race'/ethnicity

Some of the issues in relation to caring and the use of black women's labour in domestic care have already been examined. There are, however, other important ways in which 'race' and ethnicity structure care and caring. While some may be seen as pertaining to culture and tradition, others are related to the impact of discrimination, racism and exclusion.

Different housing patterns and the different age-structures inevitably affect the availability of long-term co-resident relatives among minority ethnic groups. Fisher (1994: 667) points out that research indicates that 25 per cent of Asian elders have no close relative living in Britain; that a pattern of shared care by relatives and friends may be more common amongst Asian carers; and that sons may take the lead in caring for Asian mothers (Finch and Mason 1993). In consequence, Qureshi and Walker's (1989) 'hierarchy of care' is unlikely to be relevant to the experience of many minority ethnic groups (Fisher 1994: 667). Graham reports that in one study of 400 older people, one-third of the Asian respondents and half of the Afro-Caribbean respondents had no family in Britain (1997: 129); other studies too have described the isolation experienced by those who have no family here, and no hope of family reunification. In practice, immigration controls and employment patterns have restricted opportunities for black people to live with their families and care for one another (Tester 1996: 139).

Gunaratnam (1997) reminds us that, even within ethnic communities, there are significant differences, influenced by factors such as class, migration history, gender and the disability of the person requiring care (1997: 115). The popular image of a black family, irrespective of ethnicity, is one of the extended family network; 'families within families, providers of care and social and psychological support' (Patel 1990: 36). Gunaratnam states that the most dominant stereotype of black and ethnic minority communities, and in particular Asian communities, is that they do not make use of support services because they prefer to 'look after their own' (1997: 116). His own study of thirty-three carers indicates a high level of diversity in the caring contexts of older Asian people. Some elderly couples lived alone in reciprocal caring relationships, while others lived apart from their carers; only eight of the thirty-three carers lived in extended, multi-generational families (ibid.). Gunaratnam argues that more research is needed to explore the nature and meanings of care within black and minority ethnic families, specifically the ways in which caring relationships can be influenced by individual identity, cultural prescriptions and wider socio-economic conditions (1997: 117).

Gunaratnam illustrates this by considering the low take-up of services (such as home help, day centres, meals-on-wheels) by black and minority ethnic people. Low take-up, he suggests, is not just about lack of information or lack of accessibility of services. It is also about culture and tradition; for Asian carers, the concepts of 'care' and 'caring' are, Gunaratnam asserts, highly ethnocentric. One carer in his study expressed this simply: 'I think that it is difficult for us Asian people to see ourselves as "carers" ... the idea is not something that is a part of our culture or language, it is just another part of family life' (1997: 119). There is, however, a second issue in relation to black and Asian carers, and that is how far services are inappropriate and fail to meet their specific and different needs. Most of all, Gunaratnam argues that service providers fail to acknowledge the impact of poverty, poor housing and racial harassment on the lives of black and minority ethnic service users (1997: 120).

Gender revisited

We have seen that the 1980s research on caring focused largely on women 'in the middle' (Brody 1981), on women in middle age who are caring for children and parents at the same time. Recent research on men and caring, combined with analyses of the GHS findings, suggests that, while women make a significant contribution to caring, care is not solely a woman's experience. Men (particularly older men) have always been carers of wives and elderly parents (see Arber and Gilbert 1989, Fisher 1994, Qureshi and Walker 1989). In addition, men are playing an increasing role in childcare and in professional caring capacities, working as social workers, nurses and primary school teachers (see Chusmir 1990, Cree 1996, Galbraith 1992, Pontin 1988, Russell 1983).

The qualitative research on men's caring gives some indication of the reasons why men become carers. Many men (like women) become carers 'by default', either because they have never left the parental home and a parent becomes unwell, or because a partner becomes ill and in need of care. This does not imply that they experience this caring as a burden, however. Fisher suggests that men's feelings about taking on caring responsibilities differ little to those of women: men discuss a sense of love and duty, a desire to 'pay back' the care that they have received from their wives, and to protect their children from the demands of caring. Men also report an increased closeness to their partners, and a feeling of satisfaction in 'doing what is right' (1994: 669). An excerpt from Bytheway's transcript of an interview with a male carer expresses this well (1987: 56):

INTERVIEWER: I'm just wondering if [the nursing] came easily to you?
STEELWORKER: It did. It astonished me. It really astonished me because I found I've got an enormous amount of patience ... She was a marvellous housekeeper. She could whip up a meal in ten minutes

flat honestly, if people called to the house, and that's happened on more than one occasion ... But then, when it came to be my turn, when I had to do it, I had no regrets because she had looked after me for over thirty years and I thought well she can't do it now, I have to do my best. I didn't prevaricate, I didn't think it was the wrong thing to do. I was glad of the opportunity to pay her back ... I accepted that. Put it as a labour of love more than anything else.

This is precisely the language that Graham used in 1983 to describe women and caring. It makes it clear that the ability to 'recognise the need for care, and prioritise social relationships above personal gratification' (Fisher 1994: 670) is a quality that is not possessed only by women. This is important for social work and for society more generally, as I have argued previously (Cree 1996). Ideas of women's 'natural' or 'essential' capacity to care lead to harsh judgements of women who do not live up to this stereotypical picture. They also seem pessimistic about the possibility of change; of greater equality between men and women (1996: 66).

There is one final issue to be raised on the subject of gender and caring. Ideas of a hierarchy of care have been criticised for assuming a white, Western model (Fisher 1994). They also assume a heterosexual model. Studies of the experiences of people who have HIV and AIDS have found that, for a significant number of gay men, support from parents is not readily available. Instead, care is often provided by partners, friends and the gay community, through 'buddy' schemes and drop-in centres (Brown and Powell-Cope 1992). Graham (1997) and Tester (1996) make a similar point in relation to lesbian women who seek and provide care outside the nuclear family. Tester suggests that care services are based on familist norms that promote the heterosexual nuclear family and stigmatise other family forms and living arrangements. Older or disabled lesbian women may not have daughters to care for them, but may have partners or other adult support networks (1996: 139–40).

Age

As we have seen, the dominant concern of the care-giving literature has been the burden faced by those caring for frail elderly relatives, rather than the preferences and needs of the elderly people themselves; elderly people are 'conceptualised as a passive object to be cared for' (Arber and Ginn 1992b: 87). This reflects more than a little ageism in the caring literature – a literature which has neglected, ignored and stereotyped the experiences of older people. The reality is much more complex and contradictory, with older people both providing and receiving care, and with older people choosing to remain independent and outside either informal or formal care services for as long as possible.

Arber and Ginn (1992b) point out that, contrary to the media images of the growing burden of elderly people, it is only a very small minority of elderly people who are disabled and need care. Half the population aged over sixty-five have no disability and a quarter only mild disability (for example, they need help with cutting their toe-nails). Eleven per cent of older people have severe disability and make the most use of formal health and welfare services and informal caring resources; another 4 per cent have very serious disability (1992b: 94). Elderly spouses (husbands and wives) provide virtually all the support with personal tasks for their severely disabled partners; only tiny amounts of care are provided by formal services (district nurses and home helps) and by other relatives within and outside the household (1992b: 101).

There has been a substantial increase in the proportion of older people living alone: this rose from 12 per cent in 1945 to 36 per cent in 1985. Arber and Ginn suggest that this may reflect the preferences of older people to remain independent and minimise their sense of burden on others, particularly adult children (1992b: 96). They write: 'Since the majority of physically frail elderly people are aware of how others see them, they are likely to internalise this perception of themselves as a burden, and as a source of strain to the carer' (1992b: 97).

Disability

Morris argues that the failure of the feminist researchers on informal care to consider the experiences of disabled and older people betrays the ways in which white, middle-class women have viewed disabled and older people: they have 'colluded with prejudicial social attitudes which are commonly held about older and disabled people' (1995: 71). This is in spite of the fact that disability is strongly gender differentiated: because of women's greater longevity, twice as many older women as men (14 per cent to 7 per cent) are severely disabled (Arber and Ginn 1992b: 94).

Macfarlane asserts that, for most disabled people, care is a difficult word to define. This is because 'most of the "care" received by disabled people has not been of their choosing or under their control' (1996: 13). Much care has been oppressive, often custodial in nature and provided in a controlled way. The 'enforced isolation' experienced by many disabled people is then added to by the lack of accessible public transport, discriminatory employment practices and inaccessible buildings (ibid.). Disabled people may not be able to complain about the care they receive because of fear of reprisals or punishment (1996: 14).

This is not, however, to suggest that disabled people have been prepared to accept this state of affairs without question. The disabled rights' movement and independent living schemes are examples of disabled people taking control of their own lives and making decisions about the kinds of care they wish to receive. Vasey (1996), describing her own experience as a disabled women with a network of carers, makes a strong case for the continuing use of care packages by disabled people. She admits openly that misunderstandings can occur when a friend is asked to help: friends can say that they don't mind helping, when in truth they do. Vasey asserts that it is only through paying carers that she can be in control of her day-to-day life and remain independent of those around her (1996: 87).

Mental health

There is only passing reference to mental health in the caring literature, and it is therefore to the mental health literature that we have to turn to consider the ways in which issues of mental heath may impact on experiences of care (for example, Heller *et al*. 1996, Perring *et al*. 1990, Ulas and Connor 1999). The invisibility of mental health issues in the caring literature may be seen as mirroring the ways in which mental health is sidelined in society. Clearly the stigma attached to mental health problems may make it doubly difficult for someone to ask for help. Mental health carries with it old ideas of 'madness' and 'insanity'. It is perceived as 'dangerous' and 'out of control', particularly if the diagnosis is schizophrenia, and there may be deep-seated fears about the origins and likely progression of the illness (Fernando 1988 and 1991). These issues have an impact not just on care-givers, but also on people experiencing mental illness themselves, leading them to put off seeking help and further increasing their isolation.

There are also important mental health issues in relation to care-giving itself. A major survey of nearly 3,000 carers carried out by the Carers National Association in 1992 as part of its 'Listen to Carers' campaign showed that 65 per cent of carers said that caring had affected their health. Caring caused physical problems, often from lifting and handling. But many carers reported that their worst problems were of an emotional nature. They felt isolated, angry, resentful and embarrassed by the tasks they have to perform; they felt a sense of loss for the person for whom they were caring; and in addition they felt guilty for having these feelings in the first place. Depression in carers is therefore a common experience, and this may lead in extreme cases to suicide or physical violence (Bibbings 1998: 173).

Whether or not caring has caused mental health problems in the first place, there are many care-givers living in the community who have mental illness. They may have been discharged from psychiatric hospital and expected to resume their caring responsibilities at home as partners, parents and children; or they may find themselves in the shared-caring situation of a flat or hostel living with other ex-patients. A MIND survey conducted in 1990 of 516 former in-patients of psychiatric hospitals in England and Wales demonstrates that moving into the community, while desired by most respondents, is not easy. Respondents relate that there is insufficient community care, especially crisis intervention and contact outside hours. One states that 'what is really needed is people to look after you in a home environment – people who understand and will do the basics while people concentrate on getting better' (reported in Rogers *et al*. 1993: 110).

Mental health cannot, however, be separated from issues of class, 'race', age and gender. Just as black people are over-represented in the prison population (see Chapter 7), so black people (particularly young, Afro-Caribbean men) are over-represented in compulsory psychiatric admissions (Browne 1996: 197). They are perceived as more dangerous and a greater risk, deemed in need of greater surveillance and greater control (1996: 201). Women, in contrast, are more likely to seek psychiatric help of their own accord, and women experience significantly higher rates of depression and manic depression than men at all ages (Chesler 1996: 50). Fenton and Sadiq (1996) point out that there are additional factors for Asian women here. Western cultures, they state, give a lot of importance to people as individuals. Asian traditions, in contrast, set store by people's relationship with others, and mostly those with their family and community. This means that a breakdown in family relationships is a 'threat to the roles by which individuals define themselves, and can cause tremendous mental and emotional turmoil' (1996: 254). Finally, class and age also play an important part in determining care experiences in relation to mental health: class, because, as we have seen, income and social class affects the resources and opportunities available to care-givers and recipients; and age, because of the ever-present impact of ageism (Bytheway 1995).

The politics of caring

I cannot end this chapter on caring without referring to the policy context within which caring takes place. The meaning and organisation of caring in the community (or 'community care') has changed considerably over the last twenty years or so in the UK. First, there has been a shift in the notion of community from a postwar position, where community care meant care provided by the state for those unable to care for themselves, to the position today, where community refers to 'a service provided by those people who are directly involved, not through organised collective provision' (Payne 1995: 9). This new direction was expressed directly for the first time in a government report published in 1981 that stated:

> the primary sources of care are informal and voluntary. These spring from the personal ties of kinship, friendship and neighbourhood. They are irreplaceable. It is the role of public authorities to sustain and, where necessary, develop – but never to displace – such support and care. Care in the community must increasingly mean care by the community.[6]

All subsequent legislation has followed on from this starting-point, reflecting both the wishes of care-recipients to remain at home as long as possible (as evidenced in the caring research) and also government fiscal pressures. Successive governments concerned about the 'demographic time-bomb' have sought to reduce public funding at a time when demand has been set to increase (Henwood 1990).

Community care has also been presented as a valued alternative to 'institutional' care. The impetus to remove people from institutional care is a long-standing one. It can be seen in the 1948 Children Act, which sought to replace very large children's homes with more locally based, 'family group homes' and in the expansion of fostering and adoption as alternatives to residential care for children. The critique was extended to psychiatric patients and older people by exposé of standards of care in institutions (notably Goffman's 1968 study of asylums and Townsend's 1962 study of residential care), which revealed the dehumanising and coercive nature of institutionalised care. While it is easy to agree that people requiring care would rather live at home than in large, impersonal institutions, it is important to consider again at the context in which the drive towards community care is taking place. Is it part of a move to broaden and extend social welfare, or is it to be understood in the context of diminishing resources?[7] And what about the implications behind the pronouncements on community care? Will they indeed lead to better standards of care in society, or are they intended to take power and responsibility away from local authorities, or place an increasing burden on family members (women or spouses) and unpaid or low-paid workers in our communities? Jones *et al.* (1978) summarise the issues well:

To the politician, community care is a useful piece of rhetoric; to the sociologist, it is a stick to beat institutional care with; to the civil servant, it is a cheap alternative to institutional care which can be passed to the local authorities for action – or inaction; to the visionary, it is a dream of a new society in which people really do care; to social service departments, it is a nightmare of heightened public expectations and inadequate resources to meet them.

(1978: 114)

Implications for practice

Sociological investigation of caring highlights a number of key issues for social work with adults and for community care practice. These can be outlined as follows. First, social workers must keep an open mind in their assessments of carers. This means not making assumptions about who cares (or even who *should* care), about how long people might be reasonably expected to continue to care, and what they might be expected to do. Research demonstrates that there are individual, social and cultural differences here, so the kinds of supports that people may need are likely to be just as variable. Second, social workers must be sensitive to the views and perspectives of those who receive care. This means being aware that caring takes place in the context of a relationship (which might be good or bad, valuing or abusive) and that the person who is cared for may continue to participate in caring themselves. Studies of care-recipients suggest that what we do as social workers can stigmatise and undermine those who receive care; or it can empower service users to maintain their independence and confidence. Third, social workers must take into account all the structural factors in determining experiences of caring. This means being prepared to push for additional resources (financial and otherwise) for those who are disadvantaged in society, as well as seeking to work in an anti-discriminatory way, and not make assumptions based on our own (probably privileged) experience.

Conclusion

This chapter has argued that caring takes place across a range of different contexts, both unpaid and paid, and that caring is affected to a large degree by structural factors such as class, gender, 'race'/ethnicity, age and disability. Caring is not, then, only about individual choice, normative expectations or kinship obligations. It is also about resources, opportunities and alternatives, and, as ever, it is the predominantly white, middle-class population that has access to the largest number of options and alternatives. Finch argued in 1984 for the rejection of community care and its replacement by an expansion of care in institutions. This is clearly not a viable way forward, not least because it ignores the reality that most people who need care prefer to remain at home and most care-givers want to continue to care for their relatives. But community care is not just about kin care – it is about how we in the 'caring professions' can provide good quality, non-stigmatising, flexible services which will by necessity include domiciliary support, respite care, day-care and community-based residential services. A broader understanding of caring can help us to do that.

Recommended reading

• Bornat, J., Johnson, J., Pereira, C., Pilgrim, D., and Williams, F. (1997) *Community Care: A Reader*, Second edition, Basingstoke: Macmillan and Open University (includes short articles by the key thinkers in relation to the development of understanding of care and caring).

7 Crime

Introduction

This chapter examines from a sociological perspective a subject that looms large in the public imagination. Over the last twenty years or so there has been an explosion of interest in crime. Countless books and articles on crime have been published, bearing witness to a fascination with crime that is shared by specialist academics and the general public alike. The government in the UK has devoted considerable resources to the establishment of a new research unit to monitor and study crime and crime control. At the same time, new National Objectives and Standards define the priorities and activities of agencies and individuals working with offenders in the community[1] (Home Office 1984, 1992 and 1995, Scottish Office 1991, Social Work Services Inspectorate 1995).

This chapter begins by considering definitions of crime, arguing that the definitions we use have fundamental implications for our understandings of crime, criminal behaviour and the management and control of crime. The main thrust of the chapter is on the many and varied sociological explanations for crime and deviance. I then consider the nature and extent of crime, examining historical perspectives and analyses of statistics, as well as the ways in which crime is structured by gender and 'race'/ethnicity. The chapter does not set out to review the whole field of criminology. Criminology is an eclectic discipline which draws on perspectives as diverse as psychology, psychiatry, political economy, history, anthropology, ecology, law and, of course, sociology. My concern is with sociology's contribution to the study of crime and deviance, but, nonetheless, I locate this discussion within the wider context.

Definitions of crime

The question 'what is crime?' may seem, at first, relatively straightforward, perhaps less problematic than other concepts already examined such as 'the family' or 'childhood'. After all, there can be no dubiety about what is, and is not, a crime, since a criminal act is defined as such by law, and criminals are those who break the law. But is it as simple as this? What about acts which may not be defined as criminal by law, but which we may believe are criminal nonetheless? For example, until very recent history, rape within marriage was not a crime in law, although widely recognised as unacceptable, 'criminal' behaviour. Hester and Eglin (1992: 27) argue that virtually every form of human action has in some time or place been deemed warranted, if not desirable, including slavery, non-consensual intercourse within marriage and all forms of execution.

Put another way, what about acts which may be defined as criminal by law, but which we may not see as criminal? For example, we may believe that smoking cannabis is perfectly acceptable behaviour, and we know that it is legal to buy and use cannabis in cafés in Amsterdam. More controversially, children who are involved in selling sex in prostitution in the UK may be charged and prosecuted. Childcare agencies have been campaigning to encourage the police to see these children as victims of crime rather than criminals (*Community Care*, 19–25, November 1998: 9).

Taken together, these questions suggest that crime is a relative, not an absolute concept; it is defined by society and is therefore a social construction. But there is another complicating factor. Emsley suggests that crime is 'an action defined by the law which, if detected, will lead to some kind of sanction being employed against the perpetrator' (1997: 58). There are two additional elements here. First, this suggests that an act must be detected in order to be considered criminal; and second, a sanction or punishment of some kind must be the end result for the perpetrator. Criminologists and sociologists have ably demonstrated over many years that figures for detected crime and 'invisible' or 'hidden' crime are at great variance, with figures for detected crime representing only a fraction of total criminal activity (Maguire *et al.* 1997). In addition, the nature and range of sanctions or punishments for wrongdoing are highly variable and change over time. For example, we know that in the past, the crimes of heresy, sacrilege and blasphemy were punishable by hanging. At the same time, the murder of one commoner by another was seen as less serious, meriting only a cash fine to the relatives of the deceased (Giddens 1989: 121).

This strongly reinforces the idea that crime is socially constructed; that a given society, at any time, will decide not only what is a criminal act, but also, how far it is prepared to go to police that act, and what sanctions it will impose on those who are found guilty of that criminal act.

Such a definition may be criticised on the grounds of cultural relativism. Am I suggesting that there is no such thing as a crime that we can all agree is always a crime – perhaps, for example, murder or rape or a racist assault? This gets us into further difficult areas, however. All criminal acts are open to diverse interpretations and located in specific circumstances. This means that the abused woman who finally 'cracks' and stabs to death her violent husband of twenty years may be seen as less guilty than the jealous husband who suffocates his wife in a violent rage. The same act (killing a spouse) may be viewed quite differently, and questions such as intentionality and self-defence come to the fore. Intentionality is also an issue in rape trials. When men are accused of rape, juries have to decide whether to believe the man who says he thought that the woman agreed to sexual intercourse, even if she said 'no'. As a consequence, courts find it notoriously hard to secure a conviction, especially when the victim knows the accused and has chosen to be with him in the first place (Brown *et al.* 1993). Racist attacks have also been difficult to prove, because of all the complex issues around institutional and personal racism in the police force, the courts and society as a whole (Brake and Hale 1992). (See also Sir William McPherson's 1999 Report into the Stephen Lawrence Enquiry.)

The argument so far suggests that a crime is an action defined by law as criminal and if detected, is punishable. There are a number of key figures involved in the social construction of crime: law-makers and law-enforcers; criminals and victims of crime; politicians, judges, sheriffs and magistrates, the media, police officers, social work and probation officers, members of the public and pressure groups such as the Howard League for Penal Reform. Most critically for this chapter, sociologists and criminologists have also played (and continue to play) a major role in the creation and maintenance of particular discourses around law and order, crime and justice.

Understanding crime: an overview

I have argued that crime is a social construction: that it is created by the very processes that categorise certain behaviours as criminal. From this it is apparent that the beliefs we hold about crime have a major influence on determining how criminal acts (and those who commit crime) are dealt with in society. Most crucially, our understandings about crime determine our views about sentencing, and about punishment, treatment or deterrence for offenders. Bilton *et al.* (1996: 450) locate the development of criminology firmly in the 'modernist' project: in the idea that it was possible to produce 'verifiable knowledge' about crime that would lead to better crime prevention and control. (See Chapter 1, pp.2–3, 8–9, for a fuller discussion of the 'modern'.)

The first generally recognised school of criminology is conventionally held to be the classical or classicist school of the eighteenth century (Muncie *et al.* 1996). Scholars and social reformer s at this time (including Romilly, Fielding, Howard and Bentham) set out to rationalise and codify the legal system, to make it more predictable and more effective. From the classical tradition, crime was regarded for the most part as the deliberately chosen behaviour of rational, free-willed actors: those who broke the law were believed to do so purposefully and selfishly. The objective of the law was to identify the right measure of punishment to fit the crime. Punishment was designed principally as a deterrent, to stop that individual's criminal behaviour, and to deter others from committing similar offences. There was no particular interest in trying to understand the causes or the meaning of crime. The circumstances behind the criminal act, either individual or social, were largely irrelevant to the wider project of delivering justice.[2]

Muncie *et al.* state (1996: xvii) that it was not until the nineteenth century that crime was perceived as a major social problem and became an object of enquiry in its own right. The nineteenth century witnessed widespread concerns about rising crime rates, poverty and disorder in rapidly growing towns and cities throughout Europe and the United States.[3] As concern for crime intensified, so crime became the object of more systematic investigation. The second half of the nineteenth century saw the emergence of a specialist 'science of the criminal': a deliberately scientific approach to crime which was 'concerned to develop a "positive" factual knowledge of offenders, based on observation, measurement and inductive reasoning' (Garland 1997: 31).

The new 'science of the criminal' developed in quite different ways. Some scholars such as Cesare Lombroso, working from an anthropological tradition, focused on the physical nature of human beings, seeking to uncover inherited characteristics and assumed abnormalities that might separate out the criminal from the citizen.[4] Others, using Freudian psychoanalytic theory attributed criminal conduct to serious mental pathology or at least to some unresolved emotional conflicts.

Offenders were said to break the law because of a need to act out emotional conflicts (that is, to 'ventilate'); from a desire to be punished (masochism); or because of an inability to control sexual impulses which derived from traumatic periods in their psychological development. A third area of investigation pioneered sociological approaches to crime, exploring (as we shall discover) social conditions and social factors that might explain crime and criminality. Some of the sociological approaches that developed during this period demonstrate functionalist, consensus underpinnings: that is, they assumed that norms and values in society were shared by all. As a consequence their goal was not to challenge the new capitalist system (which was viewed as 'progress'), but rather to mediate its damaging effects (for example, Durkheim 1895). Other approaches have grown out of a conflict tradition, locating crime and disorder firmly in class inequality and the workings of capitalism (for example, Taylor *et al.* 1975).

Implications for practice

Criminal justice social work and probation practice today reflect these very different and competing themes and ideological beliefs. Social workers and probation officers must critically analyse their own values and attitudes to discern where they themselves stand in relation to these arguments. They must also seek to interrogate their own institutional settings, so that they can fully appreciate the job they are being asked to do on behalf of society.

Functionalist theories

Durkheim

Writing in 1893, the French sociologist Emile Durkheim argues that crime is a 'social fact': normal and universal in all societies and at all times, and therefore endemic to social organisation:

> In the first place crime is normal because a society exempt from it is utterly impossible. Crime ... consists of an act that offends certain very strong collective sentiments. In a society in which criminal acts are no longer committed, the sentiments they offend

would have to be found without exception in all individual consciousnesses, and they must be found to exist with the same degree as sentiments contrary to them. Assuming that this condition could actually be realised, crime would not thereby disappear; it would only change its form, for the very cause which would thus dry up the sources of criminality would immediately open up new ones.

(reprinted in Muncie *et al.* 1996: 48)

Not only is crime normal and universal according to Durkheim, but deviance is 'necessary', because it performs a positive social function, by affirming cultural values and norms, by clarifying moral boundaries, by promoting unity and by providing a springboard to change in society (Macionis and Plummer 1997: 209–10). Durkheim concludes that criminals are not 'totally unsociable beings' or parasites introduced into the midst of society. Instead, they play a 'definite role in social life'.

Although Durkheim sees crime as a normal and potentially positive feature, this does not imply that he was unconcerned about rising crime in his own society. On the contrary, much of his scholarly work is devoted to seeking to understand what he sees as a breakdown in social organisation and an increase in crime and deviance. In his first major work of 1893, Durkheim examines the transition taking place in France from a rural, agrarian society to an industrial urban one. *The Division of Labour in Society* presents two very different social arrangements. Pre-industrial society typifies for Durkheim 'mechanical solidarity', that is, a high degree of social solidarity based on similar lifestyles and strong relationships and interconnectedness between people. There would be little chance of crime becoming widespread in this kind of society, Durkheim asserts, because the 'collective conscience' would be robust and effective. Modern industrial society, in contrast, is said to epitomise a state of 'organic solidarity', characterised by a complex division of labour which sets people apart from each other. This encourages a state of 'egoism', which was contrary to the maintenance of social solidarity and to conformity to law (Heathcote 1981: 347). Durkheim argues that in this kind of society, social order and collectivity cannot be taken for granted. Instead, institutions and structures have to be created to build and maintain a consensus in society (Rock 1997: 236–40).

Durkheim's distinction between pre-industrial and industrial societies has been criticised as being over-simplified and inaccurate in terms of its understanding (Rock 1997: 236). Nevertheless, key aspects of his conceptualisation of the impact of social change have been highly influential. In *The Division of Labour in Society*, Durkheim asserts that in times of rapid social change, 'anomie' occurs. Anomie refers here to an absence of clear-cut moral rules and a lack of certainty as to how to behave in the changed social circumstances: a kind of individually perceived 'normlessness' (Heathcote 1981: 347). Durkheim expresses this vividly: 'man's nature [is to be] eternally dissatisfied, constantly to advance, without relief or rest, towards an indefinite goal' (Durkheim 1893: 256). Durkheim also uses the concept of anomie in his later study *Suicide*, published in 1897. Here anomie refers not to a breakdown in social organisation at a societal level, but to an individual response to societal pressures. Durkheim suggests that in periods of sudden prosperity or severe economic depression, there is no longer any effective regulation of people's ambitions. Competitive individualism (what Durkheim calls 'egoism') and unlimited aspirations lead to a state of 'anomie', where people become disoriented and anxious, and a number of them commit suicide. Durkheim's analysis of suicide figures confirms his proposition: those who commit suicide are more likely to lack effective familial and social affiliations (for example, divorced or single people) than those who have high levels of these attachments. He writes:

> The more weakened the groups to which the individual belongs, the less he depends on them, the more he consequently depends only on himself and recognises no other rules of conduct than what are founded on his private interests.
>
> (1952: 209)

Durkheim's conceptualisation of anomie has been developed by subsequent sociologists and criminologists, who have each brought their own slant to the discussion. The idea of anomie remains popular today, and has been applied in places as diverse as housing estates in the UK and Paris, poor areas of Los Angeles, parts of Africa and the state of Chechnya (Rock 1997: 239–40).

The Chicago School of Sociology

Durkheim's ideas about social disorganisation were put into practice during the 1910s to 1930s at the University of Chicago's School of Sociology, as part of the development of an ecological approach to crime. The so-called 'Chicago School', led by Park, Burgess, Mackenzie and Wirth, took forward ideas from the late nineteenth-century social surveys which had identified the notion of 'criminal areas', where poverty, overcrowding and crime were high. They set out, through a combination of survey technique and participant observation, to chart the ways in which various areas of Chicago had become specialised around activities and occupied by the many different groups who had come to live in the city from the 1860s onwards. They argued that, like plants in the natural environment, different social groups competed for space and colonised areas of the urban environment. Their objective was not just to investigate communities, but to bring about social change. Because of this, the academics also worked as probation officers, community workers and consultants on housing and anti-poverty agencies (see Park 1936, Park *et al.* 1923). (See also discussion of Wirth's contribution in Chapter 5, pp.128–9.)

Merton

It was Robert Merton, writing in 1938, who gave Durkheim's notion of anomie a distinctly American flavour (Rock 1997). Merton argues that American society in the 1930s produced anomie or 'strain', by giving people the idea of equality of opportunity and access to success in society but then putting structural obstacles in their way which prevented them from achieving their aspirations. The 'American dream' was, for Merton, a myth, since class, 'race' and other social differences systematically restricted opportunities. Unable to meet their unrealistic aspirations through legitimate means, individuals turn to illegitimate careers instead, hence generating crime and deviance. Merton encapsulates this as follows: 'the culture makes incompatible demands ... In this setting, a cardinal American virtue – "ambition" – promotes a cardinal American vice – "deviant behavior"' (1957: 145).

Merton suggests that anomie gives rise to a series of possible adaptations, each reflecting the range of choices that are open to the individual. Apart from conformity, Merton identifies four 'deviant' adaptations (Muncie and Fitzgerald 1981: 407):

1 Innovation is the adaptation most frequently associated with crime. It is depicted as a typically working-class adaptation, leading poor people with no legitimate access to financial success to get involved in burglary, robbery and other property crimes.

2 Ritualism, an adaptation of the lower middle-class bureaucrat, happens when individuals choose to 'play it safe', keeping their

heads down and zealously conforming to rules. It is their lack of ambition that singles them out as deviant.

3   Retreatism might also lead to criminalisation (Smith 1995: 32). Instead of coping with the structural strains in society, retreatists opt out altogether and seek their own rewards through drug addiction, vagrancy, alcoholism and psychosis.

4   Rebellion is the adaptation adopted by those who not only reject society's norms and goals but also challenge their legitimacy. Their aim is to change the social system which creates the goals in the first place.

Although Merton's analysis was both historically and culturally specific, his ideas were taken up and adapted in Britain and in the United States. For example, Albert Cohen (1955) in his study, *Delinquent Boys*, points out that it is lower-class young men who are most likely to experience strain and become delinquent: young men form gangs out of 'status frustration', to gain the status and achievement denied to them in the dominant culture. Through a process of 'reaction formation',[5] they reject dominant values and turn them on their head: 'the practical and utilitarian in middle-class life was transformed into non-utilitarian delinquency; respectability became malicious negativism, the deferment of gratification became short-run hedonism' (Rock 1997: 238). Delinquency is thus characterised by short-term pleasures, toughness, excitement and thrills; typical offences are vandalism, joyriding and fighting (Smith 1995). It is also, significantly, a masculine activity. Cohen (1955) asserts that if strain has any meaning in the context of girls, this can only ever be in relation to frustrations in their sexual relationships. The allegedly small number of girls who become involved in delinquent acts are portrayed as doing so because of 'thwarted affections', not status frustration (Naffine 1987: 13).

Cloward and Ohlin (1961) develop themes from both Merton and Cohen. They accept Merton's concept of a connection between aspirations and opportunities, but argue that the critical factor here is not simply the blocking of legitimate opportunities. Instead, deviance and delinquency are based on the *availability* of legitimate and illegitimate opportunities. Cloward and Ohlin argue that lower-class neighbourhoods possess both legitimate and illegitimate opportunities for success: young men who cannot achieve success through legitimate means may turn to illegitimate means to fulfil their aspirations. Whether they do so or not, will depend on their access to these opportunities: on the circles (or subcultures) in which they are moving and on learning and opportunity within these subcultures. Cloward and Ohlin refer to this process of learning criminal behaviour as 'differential opportunity'. They identify three different subcultures with which lower-class young men might be connected (Cloward and Ohlin 1961, Macionis and Plummer 1997):

1   The criminal subculture – which is closely connected with adult crime, and is characterised by property crime, including robbery, burglary and theft;
2   The conflict subculture – which has strong parallels with Albert Cohen's notion of a negativistic, violent subculture;
3   The retreatist or escapist subculture – offences involving possession or supply of drugs feature strongly here.

Subsequent researchers have sought to test the reliability of strain theory in practice. Matza and Sykes (1961) take issue with the essentialism in strain theory, arguing that a commitment to delinquent norms is only ever partial, and that those seen as delinquent share many values with the middle-class citizen (Muncie and Fitzgerald 1981: 409). Because of this, delinquency is an occasional activity rather than a defining characteristic of their lives. Matza and Sykes conclude that what separates young working-class men from the rest of society is the high value they place on leisure; it is here that they try to recover some of the autonomy that is not available to them in school and work.

The first study to attempt to apply American subcultural theory in the British context was conducted by Downes (1966) in East London. Downes discovered that the working-class boys in his study did not experience status frustration or strain. As Rock succinctly puts it: 'They neither hankered after the middle-class world nor repudiated it' (1997: 238). Instead, they were well-located in their shared working-class identity. Neither school nor work held any special meaning for them except as a source of income, and instead they turned their energies and aspirations to leisure-time pursuits. Leisure rather than delinquency 'provides working-class youth with a collective solution to their problems'; they engage in delinquent activities only when access is limited to 'the necessary symbols of subcultural leisure' (e.g. clothing and entertainment) or when the expectation of action is met with 'nothing going on' (Muncie and Fitzgerald 1981: 410).

Critics suggest that there are a number of additional fundamental problems with anomie and strain theory. Macionis and Plummer (1997) point out that a community does not always come together in reaction to crime, as Durkheim had envisaged. On the contrary, fear of crime can force people to withdraw from public life altogether (1997: 212). Just as important, while Merton's ideas of strain may offer useful explanations for some crimes, notably property crimes, they offer little insight into other kinds of crime, such as crimes of passion. Macionis and Plummer also express reservations about the tacit assumption in anomie and strain theory that everyone shares the same cultural values, and that the only deviants to merit scrutiny are those who are poor and working-class. Importantly, they argue that if crime 'is defined to include stock fraud as well as street theft, offenders are more likely to include affluent individuals' (1997: 212). Smith (1995) offers another, equally valid objection. Strain theories, he argues, do not do well in explaining why most young men who commit delinquent acts as youths do not go on to become adult criminals. After all, he asserts, 'the strain of frustrated ambition' is likely to continue and probably even get worse over time. Yet we know that in reality, 'very few people follow this pattern' (1995: 35).

There is, however, one further issue which seriously undermines this approach. Strain theory and the subcultural studies are predicated on an assumption that the core subject is male and that the position of young women is quite different (and inferior) to that of young men. It is young men who are said to endure strain in relation to their career and employment prospects; it is young men who experience a disjuncture between their aspirations and their opportunities. Young women, in contrast, are seen as only interested in success in their relationships with men; their offending behaviour is trivial and insignificant. This, for Naffine and other feminist criminologists, is clearly 'flawed theory' (1987: 23).

Implications for practice

I have so far concentrated on criticisms of functionalist approaches to crime and deviance. There is, however, a more positive aspect to this discussion, that is, the implications for practice. If crime is, as Durkheim suggests, normal and inevitable, those who commit crime need not be written off as evil monsters or pathological deviants. This is undoubtedly a valuable message for practice with offenders. Durkheim's solution to what he sees as disorganisation in society is the strengthening of social institutions:

the family, school, religion, etc. Whatever we may feel about this at a personal and political level, social work continues to play a key role in supporting families and communities to prevent breakdown. The approach adopted by Merton and Cohen suggests a more particular emphasis. They argue for positive action policies to bridge the gap between the aspirations and opportunities available to working-class young men, through special educational measures, training for work and even the provision of jobs. Again, we may disagree with the assumption that there is a consensus about aspirations. But nevertheless the implications for practice are positive ones. As Smith summarises: 'In policy terms, strain theories suggest a progressive, redistributive agenda which deserves to be defended against more repressive alternatives; while their diagnosis may be faulty, their prescriptions can still be helpful' (1995: 36). Strain theories also serve as a counter-balance to individualistic approaches to crime and deviance, reminding us that poverty and inequality have real effects on the lives of some young people.

Interpretive approaches

Interpretive or 'interactionist' approaches present a very different perspective on the social world in general, and crime and deviance in particular. Instead of conceptualising the basic values of society as a unitary system, and the actions of individuals as determined by external, structural forces, society is now viewed as a plurality of different possibilities – individuals can and do make choices about their actions, including their criminal and deviant actions. The object of research changes to become an investigation into why individuals choose to behave in a certain way (and equally, why they do not).

Differential association theory

One of the most influential theories to draw on an interpretive framework is that of differential association (also known as cultural deviance theory). Edwin H. Sutherland originally proposed this theory in 1939 in *Principles of Criminology*, and then revised his ideas in subsequent editions of this book. The 1978 edition sets out the nine propositions which he maintains are generally applicable to all crime in modern society (Sutherland and Cressey 1978: 80–83):

1　Criminal behavior is learned.
2　Criminal behavior is learned in interaction with other persons in a process of communication.
3　The principal part of the learning of criminal behavior occurs within intimate personal groups.
4　When criminal behavior is learned, the learning includes: (a) techniques of committing the crime, which are sometimes very complicated, sometimes very simple; and (b) the specific direction of motives, drives, rationalizations and attitudes.
5　The specific direction of motives and drives is learned from definitions of the legal codes as favorable or unfavorable.
6　A person becomes delinquent because of an excess of definitions favorable to violation of law over definitions unfavorable to violation of law.
7　Differential associations may vary in frequency, duration, priority, and intensity.
8　The process of learning criminal behavior by association with criminal and anti-criminal patterns involves all of the mechanisms that are involved in any other learning.
9　While criminal behavior is an expression of general needs and values, it is not explained by those general needs and values, since non-criminal behavior is an expression of the same needs and values.

From this conceptualisation, it is apparent that crime is caused not by social disorganisation or individual pathology, but by a process of learning, interaction and communication within subcultures. Modern society is no longer seen as a homogeneous whole. Instead, different and separate social worlds are envisaged, each transmitting their own goals, and people grow up with different and conflicting definitions of, and attitudes towards legal codes. They are socialised into criminal behaviour in exactly the same way as people are socialised into non-criminal behaviour. The effectiveness of that process of socialisation and learning depends on the frequency, duration, priority and intensity of this 'differential association' (Sutherland 1939, Sutherland and Cressey 1978).

Sutherland's work has been criticised for being too generalised and for lacking a recognition of human purpose and meaning: differential association may usefully explain some delinquent activity, but it is not sufficient explanation for all crime and deviance (Muncie and Fitzgerald 1981: 416). Nevertheless, Sutherland's ideas do offer an extremely plausible explanatory framework for some kinds of delinquent and criminal activity, for example, heroin use. Most people, claims Smith (1995), have little idea how to obtain heroin, let alone how to use it. 'Even if the actual use of the drug is a solitary activity (which it often is not), it is made possible by learning what to do, necessarily with one another, often in a group' (Smith 1995: 43).

Sutherland has also been criticised for his presentation of women (Naffine 1987). Although he states at the outset that his propositions are gender and class neutral, he later admits that women do not fit the general pattern. Girls and women are conditioned and supervised more closely, and as a result, cultural diversity and anti-criminal norms are not available to them in the same way as boys and men. Naffine argues that 'the female lot ... is conceived as a state of negativity, of "otherness". Women are kept outside all the cultures of the male, criminal and otherwise. The only place women positively belong is in the family' (1987: 32). Subsequent researchers have, however, frequently used differential association theory as explanation for both women's conformity and their offending behaviour: women commit less crime because of their restricted access to illegitimate or criminal opportunities. The crimes women do commit (for example, shoplifting) are available to them in the course of their normal, daily lives; specialist tasks such as safe-breaking or the use of weapons and tools are not (Smart 1976: 15).

Control theories

Control theories have a very different starting-point to other theories of crime. Instead of asking 'why do people commit crime?', the question becomes 'why *don't* people commit crime?' Control theories have a long history in criminology; explanations as diverse as psychoanalytic theories, on the one hand, and Durkheim's ideas of anomie on the other, demonstrate a concern for the notion of insufficient control mechanisms in the individual or in society.

It was Travis Hirschi who took up and developed control theory in the 1960s. Hirschi (1969) argues that, as human beings, we have the capacity for both moral and immoral, criminal and non-criminal behaviour. What prevents us from indulging in criminal activities is neither our inherent goodness, nor subcultural grouping, nor social class. Rather, it is what he calls the 'social bond', that is, the connection between the individual and society. The social bond is said to have four interrelated components: attachment, commitment, involvement and belief. Delinquent acts result 'when the individual's bond to society is weak or broken' (1969: 16), so that there is nothing to prevent that person from engaging in a criminal act. The components of the social bond may be outlined as follows:

- Attachment, that is, the connection an individual has to conventional people and those in authority, particularly parents and schoolteachers. The stronger the attachment (and thus the greater the sensitivity to the opinions of others), the stronger the control.
- Commitment, that is, the investment an individual is prepared to make in terms of time, effort, money and status versus the costs associated with the choice not to conform. The greater the commitment, the more an individual has to lose.
- Involvement, that is, participation in legitimate activity, including employment, clubs and organisations, sport. Again, the greater commitment to this kind of activity, the less time available for non-conforming activity.
- Belief, that is, acceptance of the conventional value-system. Lack of acceptance of the rule of law, for example, makes law breaking more likely.

The empirical evidence for control theories is inconclusive. Shoemaker (1990) and Smith (1995) report that there does seem to be a correlation between strong attachment to school and family and low rates of delinquency in young people. One study cited by Rock (1997: 242) found that what separated delinquent from non-delinquent children in 'socially deprived' families in Birmingham was the extent of parental supervision (what is here called 'chaperonage'). Parents who acted as chaperons effectively prevented their children from offending, by keeping them indoors and under close supervision. Nevertheless, explanations based on control theories cannot account for all acts of delinquency, nor predict what specific types of delinquency will develop (Shoemaker 1990: 201). Smith points out a more profound complaint with control theories, namely that, because they provide no motivation for offending beyond the absence of controls, it is implied that any of us might commit crimes. Yet, Smith reasons, most of us would never think of committing armed robbery or murder, let alone weigh up the costs and benefits in doing so. Control theories may therefore explain better some acts of youthful misbehaviour than persistent and serious crime. In addition, control theories fail to give attention to the ways that opportunities for different crimes become available and are sustained over time, or to the reality that crime rates are higher in certain neighbourhoods (1995: 39–40).

Naffine highlights the lack of interest in early control theories in women and girls (in common with all sociological theories so far examined). When Hirschi tested his theory in 1964, he did so on 1,300 American schoolboys. Naffine finds this surprising: given that Hirschi was explicitly interested in why people do *not* offend (that is, in conformity, not deviance), why then did he not study girls, since females were known to be more law-abiding and conforming than males? Naffine finds an explanation for this in the strong convention in criminology of investigating the male; of valuing the male while devaluing the female, even when they are exhibiting exactly the same behaviours. Consequently, she is very scathing of studies that have attempted to verify Hirschi's ideas, presenting conforming males as responsible, hardworking, energetic, intelligent breadwinners, whereas women who conform were portrayed as passive, dependent, and 'generally lacking any of these critical faculties' (1987: 67). Naffine (1987) maintains that there was little difference between the law-abiding males of Hirschi's sample and the conforming women of later research: they were equally likely to be responsible, rational agents, in charge of their own destinies.

Feminist research has gone on to explore what Rock refers to as 'the new and intriguing riddle of the conforming woman' (1997: 242). Some of this research suggests that women's greater conformity can be explained by the greater control and supervision of women's behaviour, in the family and in public arenas. Carlen (1988) identifies that it is when domestic family controls are removed altogether, for example when young women leave home or are taken into care, that they are more likely to be exposed to controls (and freedoms) traditionally associated with young men.

Labelling theory

Labelling theory asks an entirely different kind of question to the theories discussed so far. Instead of asking 'why do they do it?' or even 'why don't they do it?', it asks 'what processes have led to this act being labelled as deviant and treated as such?' The focus therefore shifts away from the individual (and her/his motivations, family background, subcultural grouping, relationships) to the labelling agencies themselves (the police, courts, media, social work agencies, and the state in general). Labelling theory assumes that we all commit crimes, though we are not all caught. Once caught, we are not all labelled as criminal; some behaviours are ignored or are subject to a caution. The distinction between 'criminals' and 'non-criminals' is thus highly problematic, and any attempt to uncover differentiating features is, in the words of Bilton *et al.* 'equally spurious' (1996: 456).

Smith argues that the basic idea behind labelling theory was not new – 'if you give the dog a bad name, things are likely to go badly for the dog' (1995: 76). But it was in 1938 that Tannenbaum first used this idea in a criminological context, recognising that: 'The person becomes the thing he is described as being ... The harder they [agents of control] work to reform the evil, the greater the evil grows under their hands' (quoted in Smith 1995: 76). These ideas were then developed more fully by Lemert in the 1950s and Becker in the 1960s, although it was not until the 1980s that labelling theory began to have a major impact on policy and practice (Smith 1995).

Writing in 1951, Lemert makes an important distinction between primary deviance and secondary deviance. Primary deviance is an isolated act of wrongdoing, which may have little significance to the person concerned (for example, a childish prank in the classroom). Secondary deviance occurs in response to social reaction to the primary deviance (for example, the child chooses to play the 'bad boy' and sets out to annoy or upset the teacher by further rule-breaking).[6] Lemert refines the policy implications of his 'societal reaction' theory in his later study of juvenile delinquency (1971). Here he equates the large increase in cases of delinquency dealt with by juvenile courts in the United States between 1957 and 1971 with the rise of the 'rehabilitative ideal' among agencies of juvenile social control. The 'rehabilitative ideal' which had encouraged maximum intervention in the lives of young people had led to a much broader range of activities and behaviours coming under the spotlight of the social control agencies. Juvenile delinquency had, in effect, expanded to include behaviours which were not outside the criminal law. Lemert concludes that social control is a cause, not an effect, of deviance.

Labelling theory is also demonstrated in Becker's famous participant observation study (1963) of jazz musicians' use of marijuana. Here he describes the set of stages undertaken by the musicians as they learn to use the drug, hide its use from others who might disapprove, and then take on a marijuana-smoker's identity when their behaviour is labelled as deviant. From this, Becker argues that 'deviant behaviour is behaviour that people so label'. He writes:

Social groups create deviance by making the rules whose infraction constitutes deviance, and by applying those rules to particular people and labeling them as outsiders. From this point of view, deviance is not a quality of the act the person commits, but rather a consequence of the application by others of rules and sanctions to an 'offender'. The deviant is one to whom that label has successfully been applied; deviant behaviour is behaviour that people so label.

(1963: 8–9)

In evaluating labelling theory, Muncie and Fitzgerald (1981: 419) are critical of the approach's inadequate analysis of power: there is no way of understanding the processes by which labels are attached to specific behaviours. Becker's own words indicate something different. In answer to his question, 'whose rules?', he writes:

Differences in the ability to make rules and apply them to other people are essentially power differentials (either legal or extralegal). Those groups whose social position gives them weapons and power are best able to enforce their rules. Distinctions of age, sex, ethnicity, and class are all related to differences in power, which accounts for differences in the degree to which groups so distinguished can make rules for others.

(1963: 18)

In practice, several studies, both qualitative and quantitative, suggest that official labels do have an impact on delinquent identities and behaviour. Most especially, official labels affect those who are less committed to antisocial behaviour at the time the label is applied, particularly young people (Shoemaker 1990: 223). There are, nevertheless, questions that cannot be ignored in relation to labelling theory. Why are some acts and not others labelled as deviant? Does an act have to be noticed (and so labelled) in order to be deviant? What about behaviour (such as murder) which is regarded as unacceptable almost everywhere? Smith (1995: 78) points out that Becker chose a relatively safe topic for his analysis of deviance: there is clearly room for doubt about whether marijuana smoking should be considered a criminal offence, whereas more serious crimes fit much less readily into a labelling perspective. Naffine (1987) denounces the sexism in Becker's study. The jazz musicians of his study were men; women were typecast as 'squares' who held back their men from the creativity and glamour of their lives. Subsequent researchers using a labelling perspective have confirmed women's status as conforming and lacking in self-determination and purpose.

Implications for practice

Interpretive approaches, in summary, have brought back the individual into explanations of crime: they have 'humanised deviance' (Muncie and Fitzgerald 1981). Differential association has usefully demonstrated the importance of social learning in becoming a delinquent: deviance and delinquency is learned in exactly the same way that all behaviour is learned. This suggests a viable role for social workers and probation officers in encouraging young people to build friendships and associations that are not either oppositional or delinquent, through youth work and community development projects. Taking this further, control theory highlights the necessity for young people to feel an attachment or connection with the values and norms of society. This again suggests a role for social workers and others in involving young people in activities which may help to foster that commitment and increase their sense of belongingness. Smith identifies the influence of control theory on groupwork with offenders in the 1980s and offence-focused work with adult offenders towards the end of the 1980s. Control theory has also, he suggests, underpinned work with offenders' families, for example in the support given to people coming out of prison to prevent re-offending. However, it is in the late 1990s pronouncements on social inclusion that the notions of control theory seem most apparent. We can see a deliberate attempt by the Labour government in the UK to increase the 'social bond' by encouraging volunteering, 'good works', citizen participation and community involvement. (See also Chapter 6, p.123, on communitarianism.)

Smith (1995) asserts that labelling theory has had the greatest influence of all criminological theories on policy and practice in the 1980s. In spite of the fact that the political rhetoric of the Conservative government in the 1980s[7] was couched in the 'get tough' language of law and order, punishment and justice, labelling theory's two main policy implications (diversion and decarceration) were, he argues, 'almost covertly pursued' (Smith 1995: 82). During the 1980s, the numbers of juveniles sentenced to custody declined, while the use of cautions increased for all age groups. Smith recognises here a '(rare) social work success story', as social work agencies, drawing on the principles of minimum intervention and maximum diversion, turned their attention to direct work with serious or persistent young offenders, often using cognitive behavioural approaches (1995: 83). The third policy implication, decriminalisation, has proved more difficult to pursue; Smith argues that this is because there is broad agreement about acts that are defined as criminal and hence limited scope for decriminalisation (1995: 82).

Conflict theories

The third broad area of sociological explanation of crime and deviance encompasses what are known as 'conflict theories'. Conflict theories, emerging in the changing social and economic climate of the 1960s and 1970s, demonstrate a new set of understandings about the nature of crime and social order. Like traditional functionalist approaches, conflict theories are concerned with the wider structures of society. But here the similarity ends. While functionalist approaches conceptualise crime and social disorder in terms of a decline in the moral consensus in society, conflict theories explain crime in terms of capitalism, patriarchy and structured systems of inequality in society; the law is perceived as an instrument which supports and perpetuates inequality. Conflict approaches have developed considerably since the 1960s, learning from each other and at the same time taking on insights from the interpretive paradigm. The emergence of a new 'left realism' in the mid 1980s has been particularly influential for policy and practice with offenders.

Marxist perspectives

A classical Marxist approach presupposes that all social phenomena can be explained in terms of the society's means of production or economic relations (Muncie 1999: 125). Because capitalism is structured by inequality, there is no consensus in society about norms and values.

Instead, society is characterised by class conflict. The law is itself an instrument of the ruling class, designed to protect the interests of the bourgeoisie and at the same time sustain the exploitation of the working-class or proletariat.

Although Marx wrote little about crime itself, Muncie (1999: 125) identifies five key propositions derived from Marx's general analysis:

- Crime is not caused by moral or biological defects, but by fundamental conflicts in the social order.
- Crime is an inevitable feature of existing capitalist societies because it is an expression of basic social inequalities.
- Working-class crime results from the demoralization caused by labour exploitation, material misery and the appalling conditions at home and in the factories.
- In certain respects, such crimes as theft, arson and sabotage may be considered a form of primitive rebellion – a protest or rebellion against bourgeois forms of property ownership and control.
- The extent and forms of crime can only be understood in the context of specific class relations and the nature of the state and law associated with particular modes of production.

Marxist criminologists in the 1970s set out to challenge the taken-for-granted assumptions in criminology, turning attention away from individual offending to the economic structures of society (for example, Taylor *et al.* 1975). From the perspective of this 'new criminology', capitalism was envisaged as a 'crime-creating system, by virtue of the motivations which it encourages in people and the class relations and inequalities which characterise it' (Bilton *et al.* 1996: 461). Property crime was 'normal' behaviour, as people resorted to illegal means to achieve their material aims and desires. Taylor *et al.* express this forcefully:

> Property crime is better understood as a normal and conscious attempt to amass property than as the product of faulty socialisation or inaccurate and spurious labelling. Both working-class and upper-class crime ... are real features of a society involved in a struggle for property, wealth and self-aggrandisement ... A society which is predicated on unequal right to the accumulation of property gives rise to the legal and illegal desire to accumulate property as rapidly as possible.
>
> (1975: 34)

The analysis goes further, however. It is argued that any notion of 'objectivity' and 'neutrality' in criminology is a myth: that criminology has focused too much on working-class crime at the expense of crimes carried out by powerful individuals and corporations, including 'white collar' crimes, fraud, tax evasion, industrial pollution, etc. The result is that the 'crime problem' has come to be associated almost exclusively with working-class, 'street' crime, and not upper-class 'suite' crime (Bilton *et al.* 1996: 462). The solution for Marxist criminologists is to get rid of capitalism; piecemeal tinkering with the system simply allows capitalism to continue.

The period from the mid 1970s onwards has been characterised by a series of debates and disagreements about the nature of crime and crime control by writers from within the conflict tradition. These debates have been focused on a number of key issues which, it is argued, cannot be resolved by an analysis from within a pure (sometimes called a 'crude' or 'idealist') Marxist perspective:

- If crime is caused by material deprivation and poverty, why is it that not all poor people commit crime? And, equally importantly, why do rich and professional people commit crime?
- If crime is related only to structural factors, how can this account for individual choice, opportunity and meaning?
- If crime is a form of 'primitive rebellion', why is so much crime intra-class, and directed against the poorest and most vulnerable in society?
- If crime is related only to class oppression, how can this explain crimes such as racist assault and sexual violence?
- If crime is a feature of capitalism and class inequality, how can this explain the reality that most offenders are men? (Naffine states that the Marxist approach has shown little interest in the female offender; 1987: 134).
- If the law is an instrument of the ruling classes, why does it work at times in favour of poor people and against the interests of the powerful?

New studies have reworked and amalgamated versions of anomie, subcultural, interactionist theories alongside ideas of power and social control (for example, the groundbreaking 1978 study of mugging by Hall and colleagues). The key subject now is a critical understanding of the social order and the power to criminalise and control. The aim, Muncie asserts, is 'to transform criminology from a science of social control into a fully politicised struggle for social justice' (Muncie *et al.*

1996: xix). Scraton and Chadwick (1991) outline what they see as the central argument in 'critical criminology':

> Critical criminology recognizes the reciprocity inherent in the relationship between structure and agency but also that structural relations embody the primary determining contexts of production, reproduction and neocolonialism. In order to understand the dynamics of life in advanced capitalist societies and the institutionalization of ideological relations within the state and other key agencies it is important to take account of the historical, political and economic contexts of classicism, sexism, heterosexism and racism ... The criminal justice process and the rule of law assist in the management of structural contradictions and the process of criminalization is central to such management. While maintaining the face of consent, via negotiation, the tacit understanding is that coercion remains the legitimate and sole prerogative of the liberal democratic state.
>
> (1991: 85)

Left realism

Within the conflict tradition, a new 'left realism' has developed since the mid 1980s, contesting both the reputed naivety of 'left idealism' and the appearance of neo-liberal, neo-classical ideas of law and order which were gaining ascendancy in the UK and the United States (see, for example, Van Den Haag 1975, Wilson 1975).[8] 'Left realists' such as Jock Young, John Lea and Roger Matthews stress the seriousness of crime: crime has real, damaging consequences on the most disadvantaged in society. Young (1986) argues that the central tenet of left realism is:

> to reflect the reality of crime, that is in its origins, its nature and its impact. This involves a rejection of tendencies to romanticize crime or to pathologize it, to analyse solely from the point of view of the administration of crime or the criminal actor, to underestimate crime or to exaggerate it.
>
> (1986: 11)

Thus he points out that crime tends to be intra-class, not inter-class; it is committed largely by people on the edge of society, by working-class people and those of ethnic minorities who feel marginalised and excluded from society. Alienation and marginalisation lead to the greater likelihood of both petty and more serious crime (Bilton *et al.* 1996: 466). Young argues that criminology must have a practical imperative; it must address the climate of 'impossibilism' and set out to reduce crime (1986: 29).

Left realists suggest that when we think about crime, we must take on board the perspectives of all those involved in 'the square' of crime: the state, society and the public at large, the offender and the victim. Bilton sets out the three different levels of action required (Bilton *et al.* 1996: 466):

- At the 'macro' level, the pursuit of social justice is essential, requiring the state to improve material rewards, employment opportunities and housing and community facilities by fundamental shifts in government economic and educational policies.
- At the 'intermediate' level, it requires more enlightened penal policies which reduce the prison population and replace sentences of imprisonment, where appropriate, with non-custodial alternatives. It also requires more democratically controlled and accountable police forces sensitive to the communities in which they work.
- At the 'street' level, it requires environmental and design changes which reduce opportunities for crime.

Feminist criminologists are critical of the over-simplified view of victimisation in left realism. Newburn and Stanko (1994) point out that realist criminologies focus, as ever, on crime as if it were only a working-class, male phenomenon. In doing so, they lose sight of the reality that men can be victims too, and that there are very many crimes perpetrated against men, women and children which have no class basis. Crimes of sexual violence, and the abuse of women and children occur across social class groupings. Left realists have also been accused of stigmatising individuals and groups: by concentrating largely on working-class, street crime, they perpetuate the idea of the 'dangerousness' of working-class (and minority ethnic) people. In addition, it is argued that left realist criminologists pay insufficient attention to questions of social justice, because they are so caught up in questions of control and deterrence (Muncie 1999: 139).

Feminist theory

Feminist theory from the 1970s onwards has presented a powerful challenge to conventional criminology, asking new questions about the ways in which society is structured and the nature of power relations.

The feminist critique emerged in 1976 with Carol Smart's *Women, Crime and Criminology* and has since then been conducted across two broad fronts. The first area of concern has centred on the presentation of women in criminology; the second has been part of a wider epistemological project which has challenged commonplace assumptions about knowledge and theory creation. Put most simply, it has been argued that we need to recognise knowledge based on experience, and so use research methods that will allow us to understand women's experiences (Gelsthorpe 1997: 511).

From the outset, feminist criminologists have sought to expose the neglect and distortion of women in criminology. Conventional criminological theories (as already indicated) assume the male as the norm. When the female appears, she is on the edges of male behaviour, most frequently stereotyped as a sex object for men's use, or as a conforming, home-loving, colourless creature. In both situations, she is presented as a dupe: she lacks the intelligence and the power to be an active, self-determining agent of her own destiny. This sex-stereotyping is as visible in studies of conformity as it is in studies of criminality and deviance. While conformity in women is displayed as passivity and a lack of either imagination or alternatives, conformity in men signifies strength of character and positive choice on the part of men. The lack of authentic women's voices in criminology is, argues Naffine (1987), typical of the way that social science as a whole has neglected women.

Feminist criminologists have sought to redress the balance: to bring women back into criminology. For some feminists, this has meant re-examining traditional sociological theories such as anomie, strain theory, labelling perspectives, etc. from the viewpoint of women in general and women offenders in particular (for example, Naffine 1987, Abbott and Wallace 1990). Others have turned their attention to new subjects and areas of investigation, including the gendered nature of crimes such as domestic violence (for example, Dobash and Dobash 1979) and women's experience of the criminal justice system (for example, Walklate 1989). The underlying philosophy throughout draws on a conflict analysis: explanations for crime again lie in unequal power structures in society. But within this, it is possible to identify a range of feminist perspectives.

Radical feminists such as Susan Brownmiller (1975) and Andrea Dworkin (1981, 1988) conceptualise crimes such as rape and sexual violence in terms of structures of male power and privilege in patriarchy. From this perspective, crimes against women are only extreme forms of behaviours which are viewed as 'normal' for men in patriarchal societies. For example, in her well-known and highly controversial book, Brownmiller asserts that rape 'is nothing more or less than a conscious process of intimidation by which *all men* keep *all women* in a state of fear' (1975: 15). Liberal feminists are also interested in societal expectations of men and women, but their focus of attention is on gender role socialisation, not patriarchy. Oakley points to the male aspect of almost all crime, observing that the 'dividing line between what is masculine and what is criminal may at times be a thin one' (1972: 72). Socialist feminists such as Rowbotham (1973) take a very different approach, arguing that criminality is 'the product of the unequal distribution of power in both the market and the home' (Muncie 1999: 131).[9]

Just as Marxist criminology has been criticised for presenting too one-dimensional an approach, so feminist criminologies have been challenged by those sympathetic to, and critical of, the feminist project more generally. The radical feminist approach has been criticised by feminists and others for its essentialism and its reductionism; it is claimed that there are more ways of being a man (and indeed a woman) than this analysis would seem to suggest. Liberal feminist perspectives are seen to lack a structural analysis of power: there is no adequate explanation of how gender roles are assigned and why some women (including those who commit crime) manage to break free from the ties of their socialisation. Socialist feminist criminology has been accused of falling into the same trap as Marxist criminology, failing to recognise the structuring context of 'race' and ignoring human action and choice (Muncie 1999: 132).

The answer to these difficult dilemmas, for some feminists, is to disengage feminism from criminology completely: to study women 'as women', instead of trying to fit them into the restricting confines of criminology and the sociology of deviance. Cain writes: 'I am arguing that, in a sense, feminist *criminology* is impossible; that feminist criminology disrupts the categories of criminality itself' (1989: 3). The solution, for Cain, is to take a much broader approach, forefronting feminist, not criminological explanations and strategies, so that a more reflexive, gender-specific scholarship can be created. This has led to attempts by some feminist criminologists to 'place women's experiences, viewpoints and struggles' at the centre of knowledge in a 'feminist standpointism' (Gelsthorpe 1997: 522). It has also encouraged other feminists to deconstruct the language and concepts of criminology in a new, postmodern approach. Not all of this work has been done exclusively with and by women. Feminist writers and men working from a pro-feminist perspective have problematised men in criminology in new ways, examining the gendered nature of both crime and the law (for example, Campbell 1993, Hudson 1988, Jefferson 1992, Phillips 1993).

Postmodern and post-structural perspectives

It is clear from the discussion in this chapter that criminology and sociological perspectives of crime and deviance are rooted in the 'modernist' project: their aim throughout has been to find explanations and causes of crime so that intervention strategies can be identified. Postmodern perspectives see this as an unattainable goal: it is argued that we cannot make sense of 'crime' (or the family, or youth, etc.) in any complete sense, because the social world is characterised by complexity and contradiction, relativity and difference. Postmodernists therefore reject grand terms and totalities such as 'the state', 'patriarchy' or 'capitalism' as providing adequate explanations for people's experience. They also reject the idea that criminology can have any necessary theoretical coherence or unity. As Smart writes, 'The core enterprise of criminology is profoundly problematic' (1990: 77).

Moving away from 'grand theories', Foucault (1977) urges the introduction of a more historically specific analysis which examines the minute mechanisms of control, rather than concentrating on power in terms of ideology or structure. He criticises the identification of power with repression, and argues instead that power is broader than the state, and should be considered in its productive aspects as well as its negative ones. Using a Foucauldian perspective, there is no distinction to be made between 'hard' and 'soft' measures of social control. They are both part of the process of 'policing' (of managing populations and individuals) and they have the capacity for drawing on different techniques, inspectorial and regulatory, to achieve this end. Macionis and Plummer (1997) indicate that systems of control have been greatly extended and strengthened in recent years. There has been a dramatic increase in the use of closed circuit television (CCTV) in shops, motorways, and all kinds of public places. There are also more records kept on individuals by an increasing number of public and private agencies. Informal systems of control have increased too, evidenced by the major growth in Neighbourhood Watch Schemes in the UK. Macionis and Plummer conclude that there has been a major expansion in social control and surveillance in modern societies: 'Boundaries of control are being blurred and many new deviants are being "created" through this system' (1997: 226).

Implications for practice

This section on conflict theories has been wide-ranging, covering Marxist and feminist ideas as well as those of left realism and postmodernism. These different and at times oppositional perspectives have had varying degrees of influence on policy and practice with offenders. Although it may seem that the work of criminal justice social workers and probation officers today is organised largely with the context of institutional requirements and priorities, it is possible nevertheless to identify key issues and concerns that have their origins in criminology and sociology:

- It is accepted within criminal justice social work that individual explanations are not enough, and that issues such as poverty, inequality and disadvantage are important in considering crime causation and control (Smith 1995).
- Feminist understandings have had a major influence on practice with male offenders (see Kemshall 1995, Scourfield 1998, Wilson 1996).
- There is much greater appreciation of the importance of the victim's perspective, evidenced in schemes designed to bring the offender and victim together as an alternative to the 'abstract and alienating procedures' of formal justice procedures (Smith 1995: 160).
- Debates within criminal justice social work about the dangers of 'net widening' versus 'gate-keeping' (Raynor 1993, Whyte 1998) illustrate the dilemmas raised by left realists. How does social work weigh up the benefits of early intervention, preventive strategies (such as family centres, youth programmes, etc.) with the risks of unnecessarily drawing people into the social control system? While left realism and labelling theory suggest that resources should be directed to persistent and serious offenders, there is still a clearly identified need for redistributive programmes aimed at tackling social and economic inequality.

The nature and extent of crime

Two key questions remain in any discussion of crime. First, how much crime is there? Second, is it increasing or decreasing? To answer these questions, we need to know something about how crime statistics are collected, now and in the past.

Historical perspectives

Emsley (1997) highlights the difficulties in making judgements about the nature and extent of crime over time. He points out that official statistics for crime in England were not collected until 1805; before this time, certain court records were kept, but there was no attempt by government to keep annual country-wide records. When national crime records began in 1805, statistics only registered committals for trial. The system for collection was refined in 1834 and again in 1856, by which time statistics were gathered on indictable offences, committals for trial and persons convicted and imprisoned. The changes in record-keeping lead to serious disagreement amongst historians about the value of statistics. Some maintain that the figures are meaningless for serious analysis; others argue that, whilst the statistics cannot give any exact picture of the extent of crime, they do nevertheless give an indication of the pattern of crime:

> The kind of graph which emerges … shows a steady increase in crime, particularly property crime, in the late eighteenth century, becoming much sharper from the first decade of the nineteenth century until about 1850 when the pattern levels out, except, most noticeably, for the offence of burglary. After World War I, a steady, accelerating increase began again; it momentarily checked during World War II and the following decade but then began to rise sharply once again.
>
> (Emsley 1997: 59)

Emsley's own judgement is that this pattern seems to fit what is known about society more generally; it makes sense in terms of shifts in population and the economy in the eighteenth century and the concerns about the urban poor and the threat of revolution in the nineteenth century. But the picture is far from straightforward, and it remains impossible to know whether social conditions actually caused an increase in crime, or whether people were more sensitive to offences, and so reported them (and indeed prosecuted them) more frequently.

For example, the increase in burglary may reflect an increase in prosperity, because people had more possessions in their homes. Similarly, the decrease in crime during both World Wars may suggest that the police forces were too busy to attend to ordinary criminal activities; or it may reflect the fact that many young men were either out of the country or under stricter control at home. Neither example tells us anything absolute about either the nature or the extent of crime.

Emsley presents another set of complicating factors that interferes with any notion of reliability in historical analyses of crime figures: that is, changes in the organisation and management of policing. Although the Metropolitan Police Force was established in London in 1829, and larger towns in England and Wales were required in 1835 to institute local watch committees to set up police forces, there was no national system of policing until the 1850s. Before this time, a range of different policing measures was in operation. In 1856, an Act of Parliament set up for the first time a system of county-based police forces for England and Wales, with only the larger towns maintaining their independent police under watch committees. Similar legislation was passed a year later in Scotland. Emsley is doubtful about whether the new police force actually achieved its stated objective of preventing crime. What is apparent, however, is that the police demonstrated their efficiency by 'arresting drunks, prostitutes, street sellers and anyone else whose behaviour was offensive in a public place to Victorian perceptions of morality' (1997: 72–3).

There is one final development that makes comparisons of crime figures across time questionable. Emsley records that, throughout the eighteenth and into the nineteenth centuries, it was the victim or the victim's relatives who made the decision to prosecute an offender in England and Wales.[10] Emsley indicates that there were major problems with this system. Victims were often reluctant to proceed with a prosecution, because of the expense of paying for legal documents and fees, and because of fear of reprisal, or fear of losing time from work. During the nineteenth century, the new police increasingly took on the role of prosecutor, so that by the end of the century, most prosecutors were police officers (1997: 74–5).

Recent changes in the picture of crime

Maguire states that the picture of crime presented by statistics has changed dramatically over the last forty years (Maguire *et al.* 1997). He identifies four principal changes. First, the annual total of offences officially recorded by the police is now more than ten times greater than in the early 1950s. There were over 5 million 'notifiable offences' in England and Wales in 1996, compared with around half a million in 1950 (1997: 135). In addition, while criminologists in the past had only a vague idea about the 'dark figure' of unrecorded crime, Maguire notes that 'repeated investigation since 1982 by the British Crime Survey has demonstrated to a wide audience that only a minority of incidents which are recognised as 'crimes by their "victims" end up in the official statistics' (1997: 136).[11] Second, patterns of crime have changed. Crimes involving motor vehicles and offences of criminal damage have increased greatly, as have crimes of violence against the person, though these are still one of the smaller categories of offence. At the same time, there has been a 'sustained growth in public, academic, media and government attention to the subject of crime', giving access to information and analyses about a host of crimes that received little attention in the 1950s, including domestic violence, child sexual abuse, 'white collar' crimes and drug dealing (Maguire 1997: 136–7). Third, there has been a change in common perceptions of 'criminals'. While most research in the 1950s focused on male prisoners who were presented as either deprived and working-class or with serious social or psychological problems, more recent studies (for example, of child sexual abuse, domestic violence, fraud, football hooliganism, etc.) have shown that criminal behaviour is much more widespread; that 'it is to be found in "suites" as well as on the streets' (Maguire 1997: 137). Finally, there has been much greater awareness in Britain since the 1980s of the impact of crime on individuals and communities. New 'victim focused' research (for example, studies of burglary) have explored the experience of crime from the victim's viewpoint, and uncovered new information about the complex set of circumstances that lead to a criminal act taking place; circumstances which have as much to do with opportunity and chance as the pathology of the criminal. However, Maguire sees the arrival in 1982 of the British Crime Survey's investigation into unreported crime as most influential in shifting criminological attention towards victims and the physical circumstances of offences, and in altering perceptions about patterns of crime (1997: 147).

Issues in crime statistics

Reviewing what is known about crime, Maguire asserts that the '$64,000 question' – has there been a real change in the nature and extent of crime, or has there been a change in the way that information is collected about crime? – remains unanswered. Fundamental problems arise in trying to make any general statements about the nature and extent of crime.

Changes in the law and in 'notifiable' offences

The law changes over time: new offences are created and others are decriminalised. This makes comparisons across time difficult to sustain. Over and above this, the government may make decisions at times to include or exclude particular offences from official statistics, that is, to make offences 'notifiable'.[12] So, for example, the decision to include offences of criminal damage of £20 or less in 1977 immediately raised the total volume of crime in England and Wales by about 7 per cent (Maguire 1997: 150).

Changes in awareness and perception of certain crimes

A crime must be perceived and acted on as such, yet there is a great deal of subjective judgement in this, from the reporting of the crime through to arrest and subsequent prosecution (if any). Thus an increase in crime figures relating to a specific crime may be as a result of greater public and police awareness of, and sensitivity towards, that crime. Child sexual abuse and domestic violence are two key examples of offences which are much more likely to be reported and also more likely to be prosecuted today (Maguire 1997: 139–40).

Increasing numbers of police officers

The fact that there have been more arrests does not necessarily mean that criminality has increased. Instead it may reflect an increase in numbers of police officers. Brake and Hale (1992: 95) report that between May 1979 and March 1988, there was an 11 per cent increase in the numbers of police officers.

Differences in police practice

Police practice itself has a major impact on crime figures. This can be demonstrated in at least three important ways. First, the law may be interpreted quite differently in different areas, as is illustrated in the very different approach of Glasgow and Edinburgh towards the regulation of prostitution (City Centre Initiative April 1991–March 1993). Second, police records are themselves kept differently in different areas, so that some police forces may record trivial offences more than others (Brake and Hale 1992: 98). Although there has been an attempt in recent years to ensure greater consistency in data collection, Maguire reports that there are still serious discrepancies between forces which undoubtedly understate the frequency of some offences (1997: 150). Third, publicised improvements in the treatment of victims, and a greater willingness on the part of police (and indeed courts) to believe victims may have led more victims of rape to come forward, thus having an impact on crime figures (Maguire *et al.* 1997: 160).

Targeting certain crimes

Particular offences become topical at specific times, especially after a high profile incident or series of incidents reported in the media. Police forces may themselves target certain behaviours and to a large degree 'create' the 'crime wave' that follows on from their increased vigilance and proactive policing (for example, Strathclyde Police Force's 'Spotlight' campaign on domestic violence in 1998).

Under-reporting as a variable

Many offences are known to be heavily under-reported, and under-reporting varies considerably between different types of crime. Macionis and Plummer (1997: 222) identify five key issues that have an impact on whether or not people decide to report crimes to the police:

- tolerance of certain kinds of crimes (such as vandalism);
- seriousness of the offence (such as very minor thefts or brawls);
- confidence in the police ('nothing can be done');
- crimes without victims (such as drug offences);
- awareness that it is a crime (for example, some fraud).

In addition, there is known to be widespread under-reporting of crimes against women and children, including rape, assault and sexual abuse, where the victims may be afraid to come forward and face the ordeal of a public trial. Brake and Hale (1992) introduce another factor in the decision to report an offence, that is, the impact of insurance arrangements. Vandalism and theft from the person are reported in 10 per cent of cases; burglary in 40 per cent; and car theft in 86 per cent of cases. This discrepancy arises not because of any difference in perception or awareness of crime, but because insurance companies insist that car theft is reported to the police (1992: 99).

Crimes excluded from official figures

As already stated, official crime figures are related to notifiable offences recorded by the police. This figure does not include the very many 'summary offences' that are tried in a magistrate's court in England and Wales, or offences recorded by other police forces who are not managed by the Home Office, including British Transport Police, Ministry of Defence Police, and UK Atomic Energy Authority Police. In addition, official crime figures do not include the cases of income tax or welfare benefit fraud, which are dealt with by financial penalties (Maguire *et al*. 1997: 149). Official figures also exclude the very high numbers of possible offences that are reported by members of the public but which are not pursued by the police, for a variety of reasons. Maguire states that calculations indicate that about 40 per cent of 'crimes' reported to the police do not end up in official statistics, 'for good or bad reasons' (1997: 151).

Differential treatment of offences

Although most tax and benefit fraud cases do not come to court and are instead dealt with by the imposition of financial penalties, it has been recognised that fraud perpetrated by Department of Social Security claimants and property offences are pursued more heavily than more 'middle-class' offences such as tax evasion. There are discrepancies too in how courts deal with those who are caught (Maguire *et al*. 1997).

Summary

It is clear from the discussion that official statistics must be treated with a great deal of caution. It is extremely difficult to make general statements about patterns and rates of crime based on available infor-mation. Nevertheless, there are two particular areas in relation to crime that do merit specific examination, that is, gender and crime, and 'race'/ethnicity and crime.

Gender and crime

Repeated studies have demonstrated that it is men who commit most crime, serious or otherwise. Over 80 per cent of those convicted of serious offences in England and Wales (for example, crimes of violence, burglary and drug offences) are men, and in Britain, women make up only 3 per cent of the prison population (*Social Trends* 28, 1998). The most common offences for both men and women are thefts, though even in shoplifting, men are convicted more frequently than women. These 'facts' of crime have led criminologists and feminists to ask a series of questions in relation to gender and crime:

- Why do more men commit crimes than women?
- Why do more men commit serious crimes than women?
- Why do some women commit crimes, both serious and minor?

As we have already discussed, explanations to these questions have been found in both conventional criminological theories (significantly in labelling theory and control theory) and also in understandings based on gender socialisation and cultural expectations. Feminist sociologists such as Segal (1990) and pro-feminist sociologists such as Connell (1995) have sought to unpack the category of 'masculinity', to examine the ways in which ideas and structures of masculinity and heterosexuality are created and maintained. Both suggest that a way forward is to think in terms of 'masculinities': to explore the different ways of being a man, and hence the possibility of changing men's behaviour.

Other researchers have continued to focus on the behaviour of women and girls, as perpetrators and victims of crime. Wilczynski (1995), in a study of parents who kill their children, discovers that women who kill their children are dealt with very differently from men: 'When a woman kills her own child, she offends not only against the criminal law, but against the sanctity of stereotypical femininity: it is therefore assumed that she must have been "mad" ' (1995: 178). This observation has resonance with accounts of the treatment of 'troublesome' girls, that is, girls who find themselves in juvenile court for criminal offences. Hudson (1989) asserts that such young women are subject to a 'double penalty': they are 'punished both for the offence itself and for the social crime of contravening normative expectations of "appropriate" female conduct via "promiscuity", "wayward" behaviour, "unfeminine" dress and so on' (1989: 206–7). Not only this, the most common cause of anxiety at the point of referral was likely to be that the girls were 'beyond control' and/or at risk morally. The gendered nature of crime has also been explored in studies which have investigated women and children as victims of crime. Studies of rape, domestic abuse, and child sexual abuse have examined not just the experience of crime itself, but also the ways in which courts, police officers and the media have dealt with these issues (e.g. Dobash and Dobash 1979, Carlen and Worrall 1987). More recent studies have widened out the discussion of victimisation, to consider the reality that both women and men may be victims of crime. Newburn and Stanko (1994) point out that, although men in general continue to occupy an advantaged position in relation to women, this does not mean that they are not capable of suffering criminal victimisation. They assert that we must give up 'our essentialist models of gender which undifferentiatedly present women as victims and men as oppressors, and confront the social reality in which men not only routinely victimise women, but also victimise each other' (1994: 165). (Gender is also considered in Chapter 2 in an exploration of family violence; see pp.42–5.)

'Race', ethnicity and crime

Just as crime has been shown to be gendered, so black people's experience of crime and the criminal justice system is markedly different to that of white people. Marsh *et al.* (1996) indicate that black men are more likely to go to prison than white men; although 6 per cent of males over twenty-one years are from minority ethnic groups, 17 per cent of male prisoners over twenty-one are from these groups. This over-representation does not apply to all minority ethnic groups, but is particularly the case for those of Afro-Caribbean origin. The figures are even higher for black women: 23 per cent of female prisoners describe themselves as black or Asian (Maguire *et al.* 1997: 174). Black people are also, in the United States, more likely to be executed. Although only 12 per cent of the population is black, 39 per cent of those executed in the United States since 1976 have been black (Marsh *et al.* 1996: 526–7). This leads to two key questions:

- Why is the crime rate higher amongst black people than amongst white people?
- Why is the crime rate higher amongst Afro-Caribbean people than amongst other black people?

Marsh *et al.* (1996) and Smith (1995, 1997) examine a number of different kinds of explanations for the high numbers of black (and Afro-Caribbean) people in the criminal justice system. Smith begins with a warning: research carried out in London indicates that there is only ever a suspect in 16 per cent of offences. This suggests that we need to be wary of drawing wider conclusions on such a limited sample (1995: 136). The kinds of explanations for the preponderance of black people in the criminal justice system demonstrate many familiar themes from sociological literature.

Social and demographic explanations

Some research focuses on demography and social and economic factors: black people are more likely to be young, unemployed and living in crime-prone, inner-city areas of large cities. This cannot, however, Smith argues, account for the fact that certain racial groups, such as South Asian Muslims, are more disadvantaged in these respects than Afro-Caribbean people, yet have much lower crime rates (1997: 755). Smith also reminds us that time does not stand still; that there has been an improvement in the conditions of life for black people in Britain, illustrated in a striking increase in the numbers of black people going into higher education. Smith suggests that, along with such changes, it is 'entirely possible that the proportion of young black people who are criminalised will decrease' (1997: 755).

Crime as primitive rebellion

Some commentators have conceptualised black crime as a form of political resistance, a legacy of colonialism and slavery. Marsh *et al*. are cautious about accepting this kind of explanation, suggesting that black young people are as conformist to the values of wider society as other young people (1996: 528).

Criminalisation by police and the criminal justice system

Other commentators have focused on the role of the police and the criminal justice system in criminalising young black people. 'Stop and search' policy in the UK has been shown to have been used disproportionately in relation to black people, with as many as 37 per cent of people stopped and searched in London in 1994–5 coming from minority ethnic groups (Macionis and Plummer 1997: 220). Smith (1995) points out that Afro-Caribbeans in England and Wales are more likely than whites or Asians to be stopped by the police on suspicion of having committed an offence and are more likely (other things being equal) to be arrested, rather than receive a caution. They are also more likely to be charged after arrest with offences which have a high risk of a prison sentence, especially street robberies and drug offences, and they are more likely to be remanded in custody. A higher proportion of black people are sentenced in the Crown Court, and they are more likely to be given custodial sentences, rather than probation or community service (Gordon 1988). There is some research evidence to suggest that racial bias does (or did) effect sentencing by some judges in some courts (Smith 1995: 136, 141–3).

Cultural explanations

Some behaviours, such as the use and sale of illegal drugs, are culturally 'normal' yet prohibited by society. This affects crime rates for black Afro-Caribbean people (Smith 1995). In contrast, Macionis and Plummer indicate that the cultural patterns which characterise Asian communities emphasise family solidarity and discipline, both of which inhibit criminality (1997: 221).

Statistical distortion

Macionis and Plummer remind us that the official crime index excludes a range of crimes which are predominantly the province of white people, including drunk driving, insider stock trading, embezzlement and cheating on income tax returns. If these were included in official figures, the proportion of white criminals would rise dramatically (1997: 221).

As well as appearing in offenders' statistics in disproportionately high numbers, black people are at greater risk of victimisation. This is partly, argues Smith, because many are young and live in high-crime areas (1995: 145). But it is also because they experience high levels of racist attacks and racially motivated crime. Brake and Hale (1992) point out that a young black male aged twelve to fifteen years is twenty-two times more likely to have a violent crime committed against him than an elderly white woman. Studies also demonstrate that black people fear crime more than white people. The British Crime Survey found that, while just under half of Indian people and two-fifths of Black people (that is, Afro-Caribbean people) in England and Wales in 1996 said that they were very worried about burglary, only a fifth of white people were very worried (*Social Trends* 28, 1998: 161).

Implications for practice

It has been shown that we must be extremely cautious about presenting any 'facts' about the nature or extent of crime, past or present, and hence about drawing any conclusions about 'crime rates', 'crime patterns' and 'crime trends'. Criminological textbooks, the media and the general public rely on official statistics provided by the government and the police for the 'facts' of crime. But these figures have been shown to be incomplete and, at times, wholly misleading. Some criminologists have gone so far as to suggest that official crime figures are simply indices of organisational practice, demonstrating more about police attitudes and procedures than about the actual incidence of crime. Others argue that official statistics are useful because they tell us something about values and attitudes towards various forms of property in a capitalist economy (Maguire *et al.* 1997: 145). Whatever the shortcomings of statistics, it is clear that the crime that appears in official figures is a predominantly minor activity carried out largely by young men (Whyte 1998). This knowledge should not detract from any awareness on our part of the serious impact that crime has on its victims.

Conclusion

It has been argued that crime is historically and socially constructed: it changes over time, and it exists because we call it that, and pursue it vigorously. In this respect, it is always political. And crime is reflective of wider structural issues of class, 'race', age and gender: inequalities affect what is seen as crime and targeted as worthy of social control. Crime is also about individual and social circumstances: about individual choices and meanings, and about family backgrounds and social and cultural circumstances. There can be no one satisfactory, all-embracing explanation for crime and deviance, and no one solution. This should not lead us to despair. As Gorz (1982) writes: 'The beginning of wisdom is in the discovery that there exist contradictions of permanent tension with which it is necessary to live and that it is above all not necessary to seek to resolve'.

Recommended reading

* Maguire, M., Morgan, R. and Reiner, R. (1997) *The Oxford Handbook of Criminology*, Second edition, Oxford: Clarendon Press

(a large volume, demonstrating the breadth and depth of current perspectives in criminology).

- Muncie, J., McLaughlin, E. and Langan, M. (1996) *Criminological Perspectives: A Reader*, London: Sage and Open University (includes classic texts from within the sociology of crime and deviance and criminology).
- Smith, D.J. (1995) *Criminology for Social Work*, Basingstoke: Macmillan (makes clear connections between theories and policy and practice issues, although it covers Marxist/radical perspectives less well than other perspectives).

8 Towards sociological practice

In reviewing the book as a whole, a number of important themes arise that provide a way forward for sociological practice for social workers and probation officers.

Interrogate the commonplace

Be prepared to ask questions and refuse to accept 'as read' the concepts, ideas and perspectives that are part of everyday knowledge and practice wisdom. The family, crime, community, etc. are not the same for all time and in all places. Meanings change, and are created by the very discourses that name and classify the notions they describe (Foucault 1972). Moreover, the 'knowledge' on which concepts are based is itself open to question, as we have discovered in our examination of official statistics about crime. Until we have begun to deconstruct the concepts we are using, we will not understand the complexities and contradictions that are likely to affect our practice. We will also fail to appreciate the vested interests that seek to forefront specific kinds of meanings, definitions and evidence.

Think historically

Social work is frequently accused of failing to learn from the lessons of the past – of repeating its mistakes, and swinging backwards and forwards from one solution to another and then back again. Social work's ambivalence towards residential care and adoption provide two pertinent illustrations of this. A critical or postmodern outlook on history helps us to see that there is no 'continuous smooth text that runs beneath the multiplicity of contradictions' (Foucault 1972: 155). History is not a story of continual progress or gradual improvement towards a better society, or even the story of inevitable decline and impending disaster. As a consequence, the solutions we put forward today may not be qualitatively better than those of the past (as we might wish them to be). Instead, continuities and change are inevitable features of social work. I have explored this in an earlier book:

> The history of social work is not the story of ever-increasing knowledge, expertise or human enlightenment. Neither is it the story of an ever-expanding state machine designed to find ever-more sophisticated means of controlling the working-class or women. On the contrary, every new intervention in social work has been accompanied by both gains and losses along the way, and consequences which are not always expected and predictable.
>
> (Cree 1995: 10)

A historical, sociological approach encourages us to examine those 'gains and losses', so that we might make informed decisions about how practice might be organised in the future. This approach also, however, invites a degree of humility, because of an awareness that our 'answers' may be no less problematic than those of our forebears.

Locate issues in their wider social, political and economic context

I have argued throughout the book that individual experience is structured by class, 'race', gender, age, disability and sexuality. Inequality and oppression exist at both individual and structural levels; they occur between people, and are expressed through organisational policy and practice and through society's institutions (Braye and Preston-Shoot 1995: 3). While postmodern perspectives usefully remind us that there are no 'essential' categories that define people's experiences, this should not delude us into underestimating either the power or the durability of structured inequalities. The daily lives of black people, working-class people, women and disabled people continue to be constituted by exclusion and oppression. Social workers and probation officers work predominantly with people who are discriminated against, marginalised and otherwise on the edges of social life. Individual and psychological approaches to practice cannot adequately address the broader issues of their lives and experience.

Place value on individual experience and meaning

Draw on the wealth of experience that you have already, from your life, reading, films, family and friends, and use this positively to create a provisional framework through which to assess both theory and practice. At the same time, seek to discover and respect the experiences and perspectives of service-users. This means not 'first-guessing' what people feel like and believe, but instead treating them as experts in their own lives, able to bring meanings and understandings to their own lives, if we are prepared to listen (Thompson 1981).

Do not expect to find simple answers

Sociology does not provide simple answers to the complex issues of life. Rather, it provides a range of perspectives, commentaries and interpretations of social life and experience, which may help us to make informed decisions about our lives and work. Writing about the limits and possibilities of sociology, Bilton *et al.* (1996) conclude:

> We [social scientists] may not be prophets, we are not able to predict or prescribe how people should live, but we can provide a form of ever-changing knowledge that exposes the constraints and possibilities in social life, so helping people to shape their own diverse futures.
>
> (1996: 652)

This is a more optimistic message for social work than that presented by Davies (1991) and discussed in Chapter 1. Sociology may not be able to provide social work practitioners with answers, but the questions themselves lead to the potential development of sensitive, anti-oppressive practice. This leads to my final point.

Act with integrity

This may seem an old-fashioned word, but is, I believe, a useful one. It reminds us of a point made early in Chapter 1 – that all theories, ideas and practices are based on a particular set of political and moral principles. We therefore have to make choices about what theories we believe are most useful, and what actions we think are most helpful (or perhaps least damaging) for those with whom we are working. Social work is fundamentally about values and about value-judgements. Sociological knowledge can provide us with a framework for anti-discriminatory, anti-oppressive practice, by giving us the analytical tools with which to begin to explore the relationship between individuals and society, between 'personal troubles' and 'public issues' (Mills 1959).

Notes

1 Sociological perspectives

1 The word 'modern' is placed in parenthesis to draw attention to the specific set of meanings that are attached to its usage.

2 The term 'client' is commonly used in social policy and social policy texts up to about the 1980s to refer to the person who is in receipt of social work services, either in a voluntary or statutory capacity. After this time, the term is often replaced by the arguably less patronising term 'service-user'. In the late 1990s, this has shifted again, to be frequently replaced, particularly in the context of community care, by the new expression 'customer' or 'consumer'. My preference is to employ the phrase 'service-user', except where I am quoting another person's writing.

3 CCETSW's (1995) regulations for the Diploma in Social Work state that students must be able to demonstrate that they can work reflectively. This draws on ideas developed by Schon (1983).

4 Fulcher and Scott state that the origins of a scientific perspective on social life can be traced to the European Enlightenment. This marked a 'sea change' in cultural outlook, as in one field after another, rational and critical methods were adopted and religious viewpoints were replaced by scientific ones (1999: 24). The term 'positivism' was coined by Comte to refer to a means of studying the social world scientifically (see Macionis and Plummer 1997: 16).

5 This idea was taken up and developed by Durkheim in his *Rules of Sociological Method* (1938), Chicago: University of Chicago Press.

6 Throughout this book I will use the term 'black' to refer to the very many minority ethnic groups in the UK who experience discrimination and oppression on the basis of skin colour and assumed 'racial' difference. This includes people whose ethnic origins lie in South Asia, the Caribbean and Africa. The term 'black' is used in the UK as a political term. However, it is important to be aware that this has been criticised for seeming to ignore differences between black people, and for this reason it is not the preferred terminology in the United States.

2 Family

1   Hill and Tisdall (1997: 66) point out that when we speak of 'lone parent families', we most probably mean 'lone parent households', since the children are likely to have two parents in their family, unless one is dead.

2   The particular set of meanings attached to the word 'modern' are explored in Chapter 1.

3   A very similar pattern can be identified in the 1960s and 1970s as people came from the New Commonwealth to settle in Britain.

4   Hareven's research based in Manchester demonstrates that, before industrialisation, whole family groups were involved in home-based 'cottage' industries based around weaving or spinning; after industrialisation, they took their skills with them into the factory setting, where again families worked together. Kin control over factory production weakened after World War I, she argues, because of a shift towards a regime of labour surplus (1996: 30).

5   This is explored further by Macionis and Plummer 1997: 496–7.

6   British and North American 'communitarianists' such as Murray (1993) and Etzioni (1994).

7   See Elliot (1996) for an introduction to some of these studies.

8   Barrett and McIntosh (1982) are highly critical of the anti-feminist tone in Donzelot's writing (it is women who are blamed for collaborating with the new health professionals), and suggest that there is as much functionalism in his writing as there is post-structuralism.

9   This was in marked contrast to Scottish poor law policy, which sought to keep children out of institutional care and instead made use of 'boarding out' (long-term fostering) for those children whose parents were unable to care for them. Many of the children who were boarded out returned home to their natural parents at a later stage (Levitt 1988).

10 The notion of shared parental responsibility and the child's right to contact with both parents implicit in this legislation has been highly problematic for women, putting some women (and their children) in renewed danger from a violent and abusive partner. See Mullender (1997: 43).

11 This point was made vividly clear in late 1998 in the publishing of a UK Government Green paper entitled *Supporting Families*. This document called on a range of groups to work to support families better – parenting groups, grandparents, health visitors, registrars – but failed to mention social workers. The paper states that 'no one feels they are a bad parent or the family has failed because they take the advice of a health visitor' (quoted in *Community Care* 12–18, November 1998: 9).

12 Research into households headed by gay and lesbian parents reveals that there are no special problems in the emotional, psychological and social development of children (Hill and Tisdall 1997: 80).

3 Childhood

1   Children's views have also been largely absent in social work records. In an investigation of children in social work case files, Parton *et al.* (1997) discovered that children were 'silent' and their views and perspectives

were missing from official documents. Recent childcare legislation in the UK (Children Act 1989 and Children (Scotland) Act 1995) has set out to change this, stressing the importance of ascertaining children's perspectives.

2 Parton (1985) explores this in his analysis of the construction of child abuse as a problem of damaged individuals and dysfunctioning families.

3 See Colton *et al.* (1995) for a fuller description of the development of childcare services, and Mahood (1995) for an account of the 'child saving' institutions from 1850 to 1940.

4 Labelling theory is discussed more fully in Chapter 7. See also Lemert (1951) and Becker (1963).

5 My own analysis of the passing of the Criminal Law (Amendment) Act in 1875 demonstrates another such 'compromise solution' (Cree 1995: 21). Here the target was children and young people who were seen as at risk of sexual exploitation. The outcome, however, was the persecution of adult women working as prostitutes and gay men. This suggests that the regulation of children and childhood has much wider repercussions than simply those experienced by children themselves.

6 This connects with Pearson's (1983) analysis of society's fear of 'dangerous' children and sociological interest in delinquency, as will be explored more fully in Chapter 4.

7 More recently still, there was an outcry when twenty-year-old Richard Keith was released from a secure unit. He had spent nine years in prison after becoming the youngest person to be convicted of culpable homicide in Scotland. He had been convicted of killing Jamie Campbell by beating him with stones and drowning him in a brook at Drumchapel, Glasgow – not a dissimilar story to the death of James Bulger (*Daily Telegraph*, 15 January 1999).

8 See Parton *et al.* (1997) for an exposition of the worsening condition of the poorest children and families in the UK.

9 See Clifton and Hodgson (1997) for a fuller discussion of how a perspective focused on children's rights might improve social work practice with children.

4 Youth

1 This approach is demonstrated in Durkheim's notion of 'anomie' (Durkheim 1952), described more fully in Chapter 7, and in Parsons' (1949) ideas about the sexual division of labour in the family, discussed in Chapter 2.

2 It is important, however, to locate this finding in the wider political context.

3 National Service in the UK was ended in 1960; the last person finished their period of service in 1962.

4 This undoubtedly connects with Pearson's (1983) observation that there has always been a concern about the behaviour of youth and young people.

5 Feminist sociologists from the 1970s onwards have criticised the absence of women and girls throughout sociological writing, not just in relation

to the study of youth. This is explored more fully in Chapter 1 (see also Harding 1987 and Smith 1988).

5 Community

1 R. Roberts (1971: 47) *The Classic Slum: Salford Life in the First Quarter of the Century*, Harmondsworth: Penguin.

2 An example of the lack of any 'natural' support for community care is seen in the struggles waged by community members to prevent the establishment of community-based mental health projects and centres for people with learning difficulties: 'not in my backyard', also called NIMBY. (See, for example, *Community Care*, September 1994, 20–28.)

3 Rex and Moore's study builds on the work of the Chicago School, looking at the historical development of the city and identifying the idea of concentric zone theory – five zones in economic and cultural competition. (See also Chapter 7, pp.173–4.)

4 See Sennett (1980). This is also discussed in Chapter 2.

6 Caring

1 Fisher (1994: 662) argues that there were severe limitations in the EOC study's sample and its conclusions. Of the 909 replies to the 1980 EOC study, 141 reported that there was a carer in the household. Some people were excluded on the basis that they were 'only marginally affected by caring', and there was only one carer allowed per household. This left 116 carers. Despite its subsequent use in the context of carers for older people, 25.8 per cent of care-recipients were aged sixteen to sixty-five, and 11.7 per cent under sixteen.

2 The focus in this study was care for those other than children. Childcare is a taken-for-granted form of caring in much of the sociological research.

3 A total of 81 per cent of women in the UK were economically active in 1997, compared with 56 per cent in 1971 (*Social Trends*, 28, 1998: 77).

4 The General Household Survey, as part of the Office for National Statistics, asks specific questions about who is prepared to identify her/himself as a carer, what personal care and domestic tasks they carry out for others, and where this care is located.

5 At the time of writing, no figures are yet available for the 1995/96 GHS. However, the comparable Continuous Household Survey conducted in Northern Ireland found that 14 per cent of people were providing care in 1995–6. Two-thirds of carers were keeping an eye on the dependant and around half kept someone company. Just over a third of carers gave personal care while just under two-thirds helped with paperwork or financial matters. (See *Social Trends*, 28 (1998): 144).

6 Department of Health and Social Security (1981) *Growing Older*, Cmnd. 8173, London: HMSO: 3.

7 See Becker (1997) for an excellent résumé of the development of community care policy since 1979.

7 Crime

1   It is important to acknowledge from the outset that criminal justice social work, although remaining within the wider setting of social work provision in Scotland, has been separated from social services in England and Wales to form distinct Probation Departments. Debates continue in Scotland today about how criminal justice should be managed in the future, whether by local departments of social work or by a centrally organised service.

2   Criminological historian Garland cautions against using such a generic term as 'classicism' to denote the criminology of Beccaria and Bentham, and eighteenth-century thought more generally. He asserts that these reformers were not in fact criminologists (1997: 16).

3   Social surveys of the living and working conditions of the poor conducted in Britain by Andrew Mearns, Henry Mayhew, Edwin Chadwick and others highlighted the links between poverty, disease, vice and crime. There was a strong sense that 'something had to be done' to prevent the total collapse of social order.

4   Lombroso identified a number of physical characteristics attributable to habitual delinquents, including thinning hair, lack of strength and weight, prominent foreheads, thick curly hair, large ears etc. He believed that these were all indications of regression to a less developed human form – a return to being savages.

5   'Reaction formation' is a Freudian concept that describes the process in which a person openly rejects that which he wants, or aspires to, but cannot obtain or achieve (Shoemaker 1990: 116).

6   The onset of secondary deviance marks the beginning of what Goffman (1963) has called a 'deviant career'. Individuals develop a commitment to deviant behaviour and acquire a 'stigma': 'a powerfully negative social label that radically changes a person's self-concept and social identity' (Macionis and Plummer 1997: 214).

7   Smith (1995: 76) locates this in the 'political and moral climate' of the 1980s, a climate that was sceptical 'about the role of the state in promoting the welfare of its citizens: instead of being "nannied" by welfare, they were to be forcibly remoralised and made to stand on their own feet' (1995: 81). (This has been discussed already in Chapters 2 and 5 in relation to New Right ideas about the individual, the family and the state.)

8   Right realist approaches rejected outright sociological explanations of crime, arguing instead that offenders were wicked people who had chosen to commit crime: they knowingly and purposely engaged in criminal activity. The solution was therefore not greater social equality or the redistribution of wealth in society, but greater control and prevention of crime, through harsher punishment (to deter some offenders and lock others away for longer periods) and better prevention and detection measures. Control of crime was not seen as the responsibility of the state alone, since it was argued that 'welfarism' and dependency had weakened people's sense of individual responsibility, thus undermining both communities and society as a whole (Bilton *et al*. 1996: 468–70). (See also Chapters 2 and 5.)

9   Gelsthorpe (1997: 512–13) adds another three feminisms to this list: existential feminism, psychoanalytical feminism and postmodern feminism. She does not, however, go on to analyse the contributions of each to the study of women and crime.

10 The system in Scotland was different. Here the decision to prosecute all serious crimes from the beginning of the eighteenth century was made by the Procurator Fiscal, answerable to the Lord Advocate (Emsley 1997).

11 The British Crime Survey was set up in 1982 to investigate crime through a sample survey of 11,000 households, asking people if they had been victims of crime, or had committed any crimes over the previous year. The British Crime Surveys of 1982, 1985 and 1989 showed that there is a high level of crime that does not appear in the official statistics (Marsh *et al.* 1996: 116).

12 Notifiable offences are those offences that are held to be more serious; speeding, licence evasion, illegal parking and minor assaults are not notifiable (Marsh *et al.* 1996: 523). However, it might be argued that all assaults are serious and should therefore be recorded. This suggests continuing ambiguity here.

Bibliography

Abbott, P. and Wallace, C. (1990) *An Introduction to Sociology: Feminist Perspectives*, London: Routledge.

Abrams, L. (1998) *Orphan Country: Children of Scotland's Broken Homes from 1845 to the Present Day*, Edinburgh: John Donald.

Abrams, P. (1978) *Neighbourhood Care and Social Policy*, Berkhamsted: The Volunteer Centre.

——(1982) *Historical Sociology*, London: Open Books Publishing.

Abrams, P., Abrams, S., Humphrey, R. and Smith, R. (1989) *Neighbourhood Care and Social Policy*, London: HMSO.

Adams, R. (1996) *The Personal Social Services: Clients, Consumers or Citizens*, London: Longman.

Ahmed, S. (1989) 'Children in care: the racial dimension in social work assessment', in S. Morgan and P. Righton (eds) *Child Care: Concerns and Conflicts*, London: Hodder and Stoughton.

Alanen, L. (1994) 'Gender and generation: feminism and the "child question"', in J. Qvortrup, M. Bardy, G. Sgritta, and H. Wintersberger (eds) *Childhood Matters: Social Theory, Practice and Politics*, Aldershot: Avebury.

Aldridge, J. and Becker, S. (1993) *Children Who Care: Inside the World of Young Carers*, Yound Carers Research Group Publications, Loughborough: Loughborough University.

——(1996) 'Disability rights and the denial of young carers: the danger of zero-sum arguments', *Critical Social Policy* 16: 55–76.

Allan, G. (1991) 'Social work, community work and informal networks', in M. Davies (ed.) *The Sociology of Social Work*, London: Routledge.

——(1996) *Kinship and Friendship in Modern Britain*, Oxford: Oxford University Press.

Anderson, B. (1991) *Imagined Communities*, Second Edition, London: Verso.

Anderson, M. (1980) *Approaches to the History of the Western Family 1500–1914*, London: Macmillan.

——(1983) 'What is new about the modern family?', *The Family* (31): 2–16.

Apter, A. (1990) *Altered Loves: Mothers and Daughters during Adolescence*, Herts: Harvester Wheatsheaf.

Arber, S. and Gilbert, N. (1989) 'Men: The forgotten carers', *Sociology* 23 (1): 111–18.

Arber, S. and Ginn, J. (1991) *Gender and Later Life: A Sociological Analysis of Resources and Constraints*, London: Sage.

——(1992a) 'Class and caring: a forgotten dimension', *Sociology* 26: 619–34.

——(1992b) ' "In sickness and in health": care-giving, gender and the independence of elderly people', in C. Marsh and S. Arber (eds) *Families and Households: Divisions and Change*, Basingstoke: Macmillan.

Archard, D. (1993) *Children: Rights and Childhood*, London: Routledge.

Aries, P. (1962) *Centuries of Childhood*, London: Jonathan Cape.

Bailey, R. and Brake, M. (1975) *Radical Social Work*, London: Edward Arnold.

Baker Miller, J. (1978) *Towards a New Psychology for Women*, London: Pelican.

Baldwin, D., Coles, B. and Mitchell, W. (1997) 'The formation of an underclass or disparate processes of social exclusion? Evidence from two groupings of "vulnerable youth" ', in R. MacDonald (ed.) *Youth, the 'Underclass' and Social Exclusion*, London: Routledge.

Ball, D.W. (1974) 'The family as a sociological problem', in A. Skolnick and J. Skolnick (eds) *Intimacy, Family and Society*, Boston: Little, Brown.

Banks, M., Bates, I., Breakwell, G., Brynner, J., Emler, N., Jamieson, L. and Roberts, K. (1992) *Careers and Identities*, Buckingham: Open University Press.

Banton, M. (1965) *Roles: An Introduction to the Study of Social Relations*, London: Tavistock.

Barclay Committee (1982) *Social Workers: Their Roles and Tasks*, London: Bedford Square Press.

Barn, R. (1993) *Black Children in the Public Child Care System*, London: Batsford.

Barrett, M. and McIntosh, M. (1982) *The Anti-Social Family*, London: Verso.

Bauman, Z. (1990) *Thinking Sociologically*, Oxford: Basil Blackwell.

——(1992) *Intimations of Modernity*, London: Routledge.

Becker, H. (1963) *Outsiders*, New York: Free Press.

Becker, S. (1997) *Responding to Poverty: The Politics of Cash and Care*, London: Longman.

Becker, S., Aldridge, J. and Deardon, C. (1998) *Young Carers and their Families*, Oxford: Blackwell.

Beechey, V. (1986) 'Familial ideology', in V. Beechey and J. Donald (eds) *Subjectivity and Social Relations*, Milton Keynes: Open University Press.

——(1987) *Unequal Work*, London: Verso.

Beechey, V. and Perkins, T. (1987) *A Matter of Hours: Women, Part-time Work and the Labour Market*, Cambridge: Polity Press.

Bell, C. (1968) *Middle Class Families*, London: Routledge and Kegan Paul.

Bell, C. and Newby, H. (1971) *Community Studies*, London: Allen and Unwin.

——(1976) 'Community, communion, class and community action: the social sources of the new urban politics', in D.J. Herbert and R.J. Johnson (eds), *Social Areas in Cities*, London: Wiley.

Berger, P.L. (1967) *Invitation to Sociology: A Humanist Perspective*, Harmondsworth: Penguin.

Berger, P.L. and Kellner, H. (1971) 'Marriage and the construction of reality', in B.R. Cosin (ed.) *School and Society*, London: Routledge and Kegan Paul.

Berger, P.L. and Luckman, T. (1967) *The Social Construction of Reality*, Harmondsworth: Penguin.

Bernard, J. (1972) *The Future of Marriage*, New York: Bantam.

Bernardes, J. (1997) *Family Studies: An Introduction*, London: Routledge.

Bhavnani, K. and Coulson, M. (1986) 'Transforming socialist-feminism: The challenge of racism', *Feminist Review* 23: 81–92.

Bibbings, A. (1998) 'Carers and professionals – the carer's viewpoint', in M. Allott and M. Robb (eds) *Understanding Health and Social Care: An Introductory Reader*, London: Sage and the Open University.

Bilton, T., Bonnett, K., Jones, P., Skinner, D., Stanworth, M. and Webster, A. (1996) *Introducing Sociology*, Third edition, Basingstoke: Macmillan.

Black, D. and Cottrell, D. (1993) *Seminars in Child and Adolescent Psychiatry*, London: Gaskell.

Blau, P.M. (1964) *Exchange and Power in Social Life*, New York: Wiley.

Bornat, J., Johnson, J., Pereira, C., Pilgrim, D. and Williams, F. (1997) *Community Care: A Reader*, Second edition, Basingstoke: Macmillan and Open University.

Boyden, J. (1990) 'Childhood and the policy makers: a comparative perspective on the globalization of childhood', in A. James and A. Prout (eds) *Constructing and Reconstructing Childhood: Contemporary Issues in the Sociological Study of Childhood*, London: Falmer Press.

Brake, M. and Hale, C. (1992) *Public Order and Private Lives: The Politics of Law and Order*, London: Routledge.

Braye, S. and Preston-Shoot, M. (1995) *Empowering Practice in Social Care*, Buckingham: Open University Press.

Brittan, A. and Maynard, M. (1984) *Sexism, Racism and Oppression*, Oxford: Basil Blackwell.

Brody, E.M. (1981) 'Women in the middle and family help to older people', *The Gerontologist* 21: 471–80.

Brook, E. and Davis, A. (eds) (1985) *Women, the Family and Social Work*, London: Tavistock.

Brown, B., Burman, M. and Jamieson, L. (1993) *Sex Crimes on Trial,* Edinburgh: Edinburgh University Press.

Brown, M.A. and Powell-Cope, G.M. (1992) *Caring for a Loved-One with AIDS*, Seattle, WA: University of Washington.

Browne, D. (1996) 'The black experience of mental health law', in T. Heller, J. Reynolds, R. Gomm, R. Muston and S. Pattison (eds) *Mental Health Matters: A Reader*, Basingstoke: Macmillan, in association with the Open University.

Browne, J. (1995) 'Can social work empower?', in R. Hugman and D. Smith (eds) *Ethical Issues in Social Work*, London: Routledge.

Brownmiller, S. (1975) *Against Our Will: Men, Women and Rape*, Harmondsworth: Penguin.

Bryan, A. (1992) 'Working with black single mothers: myths and reality', in M. Langan and L. Day (eds) *Women, Oppression and Social Work*, London: Routledge.

Bulmer, M. (1987) *The Social Basis of Community Care*, London: Allen and Unwin.

Bytheway, B. (1987) *Informal Care Systems: an Exploratory Study within the Families of Older Steel Workers in South Wales*, York: Joseph Rowntree Memorial Trust.

——(1995) *Ageing*, Buckingham: Open University Press.

Cain, M. (1989) *Growing up Good: Policing the Behaviour of Girls in Europe*, London: Sage.

Campbell, A. (1981) *Delinquent Girls*, Oxford: Blackwell.

Campbell, B. (1993) *Goliath: Britain's Dangerous Places*, London: Methuen.

Cannan, C. (1992) *Changing Families: Changing Welfare*, Hemel Hempstead: Harvester Wheatsheaf.

Cannan, C. and Warren, C. (1997) *Social Action with Children and Families: A Community Development Approach to Child and Family Welfare*, London: Routledge.

Carlen, P. (1988) *Women, Crime and Poverty*, Milton Keynes: Open University Press.

——(1992) 'Criminal women and criminal justice: the limits to, and potential of, feminist and left realist perspectives', in R. Matthews and J. Young (eds) *Issues in Realist Criminology*, London: Sage.

Carlen, P. and Worrall, A. (1987) *Gender, Crime and Justice*, Milton Keynes: Open University Press.

Cavanagh, K. and Cree, V.E. (eds) (1996) *Working with Men: Feminism and Social Work*, London: Routledge.

Central Council for Education and Training in Social Work (1995) *Assessing for Quality: Rules and Requirements for the Diploma in Social Work*, London: CCETSW.

Cheal, D. (1991) *Family and the State of Theory*, Hemel Hempstead: Harvester Wheatsheaf.

Chesler, P. (1996) 'Women and madness: the mental asylum', in T. Heller, J. Reynolds, R. Gomm, R. Muston and S. Pattison (eds) *Mental Health Matters: A Reader*, Basingstoke: Macmillan, in association with the Open University.

Chester, R. (1985) 'The rise of the neo-conventional family', *New Society* (9 May), 185–8.

Chisholm, L. and Du Bois-Reymond, M. (1993) 'Youth transitions, gender and social change', *Sociology* 27 (2): 259–79.

Chisholm, L., Brown, P., Buchner, P. and Kruger, H. (1990) 'Childhood and youth studies in the United Kingdom and West Germany: an introduction', in L. Chisholm, P. Buchner, H. Kruger and P. Brown (eds) *Childhood, Youth and Social Change: A Comparative Perspective*, London: Falmer Press.

Chodorow, N.J. (1978) *The Reproduction of Mothering*, Berkeley: University of California Press.

——(1989) *Feminism and Psychoanalytic Theory*, London: Yale University Press.

Chusmir, L.C. (1990) 'Men who make non-traditional career choices', *Journal of Counseling and Development* 69: 11–16.

City Centre Initiative (April 1991–March 1993) *Out in the Cold*, Glasgow: City Centre Initiative.

Clarke, J., Hall, S., Jefferson, T. and Roberts, B. (1976) 'Subcultures, cultures and class', in S. Hall and T. Jefferson (eds) *Resistance through Rituals: Youth Subcultures in Post-War Britain*, London: Hutchinson and CCCS, University of Birmingham.

Clarke, L. (1995) 'Family care and changing family structure: bad news for the elderly?', in I. Allen and E. Perkins (eds) *The Future of Family Care for Older People*, London: HMSO.

Clifton, J. and Hodgson, D. (1997) 'Rethinking practice through a children's rights perspective', in C. Cannan and C. Warren (eds) *Social Action with Children and Families: A Community Development Approach to Child and Family Welfare*, London: Routledge.

Cloward, R. and Ohlin, L. (1961) *Delinquency and Opportunity: a Theory of Delinquent Gangs*, London: Routledge and Kegan Paul.

Cohen, A. (1955) *Delinquent Boys: The Culture of the Gang*, Chicago: Free Press.

Cohen, S. (1972) *Folk Devils and Moral Panics: The Creation of Mods and Rockers*, Oxford: Martin Robertson.

——(1985) *Visions of Social Control: Crime, Punishment and Classification*, Cambridge: Polity Press.

Coleman, J.C. (1979) *The School Years*, London: Methuen.

——(1990) *The Nature of Adolescence*, Second edition, London: Routledge.

——(1992) 'The nature of adolescence', in J.C. Coleman and C. Warren-Adamson (eds) *Youth Policy in the 1990s: The Way Forward*, London: Routledge.

Colton, M., Drury, C. and Williams, M. (1995) *Children in Need: Family Support under the Children Act 1989*, Aldershot: Avebury.

Connell, R.W. (1983) *Which Way is Up?* London: Allen and Unwin.

——(1995) *Masculinities*, Cambridge: Polity Press.

Cooper, D. (1971) *Death of the Family*, London: Allen Lane.

Cornwell, J. (1984) *Hard-earned Lives: Accounts of Health and Illness from East London*, London: Tavistock.

Cree, V.E. (1995) *From Public Streets to Private Lives: The Changing Task of Social Work*, Aldershot: Avebury.

——(1996) 'Why do men care?', in K. Cavanagh and V.E. Cree (eds) *Working with Men: Feminism and Social Work*, London: Routledge.

Cross, W. E. (1971) 'The Negro to black conversion experience: towards the psychology of black liberation', *Black World* 20: 13–27.

Dahrendorf, R. (1957) *Class and Class Conflict in an Industrial Society*, London: Routledge and Kegan Paul.

Dalley, G. (1988) *Ideologies of Caring*, Basingstoke: Macmillan.

Davies, J. (1993) 'Introduction', in J. Davies, B. Berger and A.Carlson (eds) *The Family: Is It Just Another Lifestyle Choice?*, London: Institute of Economic Affairs, Health and Welfare Unit.

Davies, J., Berger, B. and Carlson, A. (eds) *The Family: Is It Just Another Lifestyle Choice?*, London: Institute of Economic Affairs, Health and Welfare Unit.

Davies, M. (ed.) (1991) *The Sociology of Social Work*, London: Routledge.

Davis, H. and Bourhill, M. (1997) ' "Crisis": the demonization of children and young people', in P. Scraton (ed.) *'Childhood' in 'Crisis'?*, London: UCL Press.

Davis, J. (1990) *Youth and the Condition of Britain*, London: Athlone Press.

Davis, K. (1996) 'Disability and legislation: rights and equality', in G. Hales (ed.) *Beyond Disability: Towards an Enabling Environment*, London: Sage, in association with the Open University.

Davis, L. (ed.) (1997) *Disability Studies: A Reader*, London: Routledge.

Day, P.R. (1987) *Sociology in Social Work Practice*, Basingstoke: Macmillan.

Delphy, C. (1984) *Close to Home: A Materialist Analysis of Women's Oppression*, London: Hutchinson.

Delphy, C. and Leonard, D. (1992) *Familiar Exploitation: A New Analysis of Marriage in Contemporary Western Societies*, Cambridge: Polity Press.

Dennis, N. and Erdos, G. (1993) *Families without Fatherhood*, Second edition, London: Institute of Economic Affairs, Health and Welfare Unit.

Dennis, R. and Daniels, S. (1996) ' "Community" and the social geography of Victorian cities', in M. Drake (ed.) *Time, Family and Community: Perspectives on Family and Community History*, Oxford: Blackwell.

Denzin, N.K. (1987) 'Post modern children', *Society* 24 (3): 32–5.

Department of Health (1995) *Child Protection: Messages from Research*, London: HMSO.

Dingwall, R., Eekelaar, J. and Murray, T. (1983; Second edn 1995) *The Protection of Children: State Intervention and Family Life*, Aldershot: Avebury.

Dobash, R.E. and Dobash, R.P. (1979) *Violence against Wives: a Case Against Patriarchy*, New York: Free Press.

——(eds) (1992) *Women, Violence and Social Change*, London: Routledge.

Dominelli, L. (1997) *Sociology for Social Work*, Basingstoke: Macmillan.

Dominelli, L. and McLeod, E. (1989) *Feminist Social Work*, Basingstoke: Macmillan.

Donzelot, J. (1980) *The Policing of Families*, London: Hutchinson.

Downes, D. (1966) *The Delinquent Solution*, London: Routledge and Kegan Paul.

Durkheim, E. (1893, 1984) *The Division of Labour in Society*, London: Macmillan.

——(1895, 1982) *The Rules of the Sociological Method*, London: Macmillan.

——(1952) *Suicide: A Study in Sociology*, London: Routledge and Kegan Paul.

Dworkin, A. (1981) *Pornography: Men Possessing Women*, London: Women's Press.

——(1988) *Letters from A War Zone: Writings 1976–1987*, London: Secker and Warburg.

Eisenstadt, S.N. (1956) *From Generation to Generation*, New York: The Free Press.

Elliot, F.R. (1996) *Gender, Family and Society*, Basingstoke: Macmillan.

Emsley, C. (1997) 'The history of crime and crime control institutions', in M. Maguire, R. Morgan and R. Reiner (eds) *The Oxford Handbook of Criminology*, Second edition, Oxford: Clarendon Press.

Engels, F. (1902) *The Origin of the Family, Private Property and the State*, Chicago: Charles H. Kerr and Company.

Ennew, J. (1986) *The Sexual Exploitation of Children*, Oxford: Basil Blackwell.

——(1994) 'Time for children or time for adults?', in J. Qvortrup, M. Bardy, G. Sgritta and H. Wintersberger (eds) *Childhood Matters: Social Theory, Practice and Politics*, Aldershot: Avebury.

Epstein, J.S. (1998) *Youth Culture: Identity in a Postmodern World*, Oxford: Blackwell.

Equal Opportunities Commission (1980) *The Experience of Caring for Elderly and Handicapped Dependants: Survey Report*, Manchester: EOC.

——(1982) *Caring for the Elderly and Handicapped: Community Care Policies and Women's Lives*, Manchester: EOC.

Erikson, E. (1968) *Identity: Youth and Crisis*, London: Faber.

Etzioni, A. (1994) *The Spirit of Community: Rights, Responsibilities and the Communitarian Agenda*, New York: Simon and Schuster.

Evandrou, M. (1990) *Challenging the Invisibility of Carers: Mapping Informal Care Nationally*, WSP/49, London: STICERD.

Evans, K. and Fraser, P. (1996) 'Difference in the city: locating marginal use of public space', in C. Samson and N. South (eds) *The Social Construction of Social Policy: Methodologies, Racism, Citizenship and the Environment*, Basingstoke: Macmillan.

Fawcett, B., Featherstone, B., Hearn, J. and Toft, C. (eds) (1996) *Violence and Gender Relations: Theories and Interventions*, London: Sage

Featherstone, B. and Fawcett, B. (1995) 'Oh no! not more isms: feminism, post-modernism, post-structuralism and social work education', *Social Work Education* 14 (3): 25–43.

Fenton, S. and Sadiq, A. (1996) 'Asian women speak out', in T. Heller, J. Reynolds, R. Gomm, R. Muston and S. Pattison (eds) *Mental Health Matters: A Reader*, Basingstoke: Macmillan, in association with the Open University.

Fernando, S. (1988) *Race and Culture in Psychiatry*, London: Croom Helm.

——(1991) *Mental Health, Race and Culture*, London: MIND.

——(ed.) (1995) *Mental Health in a Multi-Ethnic Society: A Multi-disciplinary Handbook*, London: Routledge.

Ferri, E. and Smith, K. (1996) *Parenting in the 1990s*, London: Family Policy Studies Centre and Joseph Rowntree Foundation.

Finch, J. (1984) 'Community care: Developing non-sexist alternatives', *Critical Social Policy* 9 (Spring): 6–18.

——(1989) *Family Obligations and Social Change*, London: Polity Press.

——(1995) 'Responsibilities, obligations and commitments', in I. Allen and E. Perkins (eds) *The Future of Family Care for Older People*, London: HMSO.

Finch, J. and Groves, D. (1980) 'Community care and the family: a case for equal opportunities', *Journal of Social Policy* 9 (4): 487–511.

Finch, J. and Mason, J. (1993) *Negotiating Family Responsibilities*, London: Routledge.

Fischer, J. (1978) *Effective Casework Practice*, New York: McGraw-Hill.

Fisher, M. (1994) 'Man-made care: Community care and older male carers', *British Journal of Social Work* (24): 659–80.

——(1997) 'Older male carers and community care', in J. Bornat, J. Johnson, C. Pereira, D. Pilgrim and F. Williams (eds) *Community Care: A Reader*, Second edition, Basingstoke: Macmillan and Open University.

Fletcher, R. (1973) *The Family and Marriage in Britain*, Harmondsworth: Penguin.

Foster, J. (1996) ' "Island homes for island people": competition, conflict and racism in the battle over public housing on the Isle of Dogs', in C. Samson and N. South (eds) *The Social Construction of Social Policy: Methodologies, Racism, Citizenship and the Environment*, Basingstoke: Macmillan.

Foucault, M. (1972) *The Archaeology of Knowledge*, London: Tavistock.

——(1977) *Discipline and Punish*, London: Allen Lane.

Freud, A. (1937) *The Ego and the Mechanisms of Defence*, London: Hogarth Press.

——(1958) 'Adolescence', *Psychoanalytical Study of the Child* 13: 255–78.

Frones, I. (1994) 'Dimensions of childhood', in J. Qvortrup, M. Bardy, G. Sgritta and H. Wintersberger (eds) *Childhood Matters: Social Theory, Practice and Politics*, Aldershot: Avebury.

Frost, N. and Stein, M. (1989) *The Politics of Child Welfare: Inequality, Power and Change*, Hemel Hempstead: Harvester Wheatsheaf.

Fulcher, J. and Scott, J. (1999) *Sociology*, Oxford: Oxford University Press.

Galbraith, M. (1992) 'Understanding career choices of men in elementary education', *Journal of Educational Research* 85 (4): 246–53.

Gans, H.J. (1980) 'Urbanism and suburbanism as ways of life (1968)', in R. Bocock, P. Hamilton, K. Thompson and A. Waton (eds) *An Introduction to Sociology*, London: Fontana.

Garfinkel, H. (1967) *Studies in Ethnomethodology*, Englewood Cliffs, NJ: Prentice Hall.

Garland, D. (1997) 'Of crimes and criminals: the development of criminology in Britain', in M. Maguire, R. Morgan and R. Reiner (eds) *The Oxford Handbook of Criminology*, Second edition, Oxford: Clarendon Press.

Garratt, D. (1997) 'Youth cultures and subcultures', in J. Roche and S. Tucker (eds) *Youth in Society*, London: Open University and Sage.

Gelles, R.J. (1979) *Family Violence*, London, Sage.

Gelsthorpe, L. (1997) 'Feminism and criminology', in M. Maguire, R. Morgan and R. Reiner (eds) *The Oxford Handbook of Criminology*, Second edition, Oxford: Clarendon Press.

Giddens, A. (1982) *Sociology: A Brief but Critical Introduction*, Basingstoke: Macmillan.

——(1989) *Sociology*, Cambridge: Polity Press.

Gilligan, C. (1982) *In a Different Voice: Psychological Theory and Women's Development*, Cambridge, Mass.: Harvard University Press.

Gillis, J.R. (1981) *Youth and History: Tradition and Change in European Age Relations, 1770–Present*, New York: Academic Press.

Gilroy, P. (1992) 'The end of anti-racism', in J. Donald and A. Rattansi (eds) *'Race', Culture and Difference*, London: Sage.

Gittins, D. (1993) *The Family in Question: Changing Households and Familiar Ideologies*, Second edition, Basingstoke: Macmillan.

——(1998) *The Child in Question*, Basingstoke: Macmillan.

Glendinning, C. (1992) *The Costs of Informal Care*, London: HMSO.

Goffman, E. (1963) *Stigma: Notes on the Management of Spoiled Identity*, Englewood Cliffs, NJ: Prentice Hall.

——(1968) *Asylums: Essays on the Social Situation of Mental Patients and Other Inmates*, London: Penguin.

——(1969) *The Presentation of Self in Everyday Life*, Harmondsworth: Penguin.

Gordon, L. (1988) *Heroes of Their Own Lives: The Politics and History of Family Violence, Boston 1880–1960*, London: Virago.

Gordon, P. (1988) 'Black people and the criminal law: rhetoric and reality', *International Journal of the Sociology of Law* 16 (3).

Gorz, A. (1982) *Farewell to the Working Class*, London: Pluto.

Graham, H. (1983) 'Caring: a labour of love', in J. Finch and D. Groves (eds) *A Labour of Love: Women, Work and Caring*, London: Routledge and Kegan Paul.

——(1991) 'The concept of caring in feminist research: the case of domestic service', *Sociology* 25 (1): 61–78.

——(1997) 'Feminist perspectives on caring', in J. Bornat, J. Johnson, C. Pereira, D. Pilgrim and F. Williams (eds) *Community Care: A Reader*, Second edition, Basingstoke: Macmillan and Open University.

Gramsci, A. (1971) *Selections for the Prison Notebooks*, London: New Left Books.

Grbich, C. (1990) 'Socialisation and social change: a critique of three positions', *British Journal of Sociology* 41 (4): 517–30.

Green, H. (1988) *Informal Carers*, Series GHS No. 15, London: HMSO.

Gregson, N. and Lowe, M. (1994) *Servicing the Middle Classes*, London: Routledge.

Griffiths, V. (1995) *Adolescent Girls and Their Friends: A Feminist Ethnography*, Aldershot: Avebury.

Gubrium, J.F. and Silverman, D. (1989) *The Politics of Field Research*, London: Sage.

Gunaratnam, Y. (1997) 'Breaking the silence: black and ethnic minority carers and service provision', in J. Bornat, J. Johnson, C. Pereira, D. Pilgrim and F. Williams (eds) *Community Care: A Reader*, Second edition, Basingstoke: Macmillan and Open University.

Habermas, J. (1981a) *The Theory of Communicative Action*, i: *Reason and the Rationalisation of Society*, London: Heinemann.

——(1981b) *The Theory of Communicative Action*, ii: *The Critique of Functionalist Reason*, London: Heinemann.

Hall, G.S. (1904) *Adolescence: Its Psychology and its Relations to Physiology, Anthropology, Sociology, Sex, Crime, Religion and Education*, New York: Appleton.

Hall, S. (1991) 'The local and the global: globalisation and ethnicity', in A. King (ed.) *Culture, Globalisation and the World-System*, Basingstoke: Macmillan.

Hall, S., and Jefferson, T. (eds) (1976) *Resistance through Rituals: Youth Subcultures on Post-War Britain*, London: Hutchinson.

Hall, S., Critcher, C., Jefferson, T., Clarke, J. and Roberts, B. (1978) *Policing the Crisis: Mugging, the State and Law and Order*, Basingstoke: Macmillan.

Hallett, C. (1993) 'Child protection in Europe: convergence or divergence?', *Adoption and Fostering*, 17 (4): 27–32.

Hanmer, J. and Statham, D. (1988, 2001) *Women and Social Work: Towards a Woman-Centred Practice*, Basingstoke: Macmillan.

Hardiker, P. and Barker, M. (1981) *Theories of Practice in Social Work*, London: Academic Press.

Harding, S. (1987) *Feminism and Methodology*, Milton Keynes: Open University Press.

——(1991) *Whose Science? Whose Knowledge? Thinking from Women's Lives*, Milton Keynes: Open University Press.

Hareven, T.K. (1996) 'Recent research on the history of the family', in M. Drake (ed.) *Time, Family and Community: Perspectives on Family and Community History*, Oxford: Blackwell.

Harris, R. (1989) 'Child protection, child care and child welfare', in K. Wilson and A. James (eds) *The Child Protection Handbook*, Hemel Hempstead: Harvester Wheatsheaf.

Hartmann, H. (1981) 'The family as the locus of gender, class and political struggle', *Signs* 6: 366–94.

Harvey, D. (1973) *Social Justice and the City*, London: Edward Arnold.

Harvey, L. (1990) *Critical Social Research*, London: Unwin Hyman.

Hearn, J. (1996) 'The origins of violence: men, gender relations, organisations and violences', in B. Fawcett, B. Featherstone, J. Hearn and C. Toft (eds) *Violence and Gender Relations: Theories and Interventions*, London: Sage.

Hearn, J. and Parkin, W. (1987) *Sex at Work: The Power and Paradox of Organisational Sexuality*, Brighton: Wheatsheaf.

Heathcote, F. (1981) 'Social disorganisation theories', in M. FitzGerald, G. McLennan and J. Pawson (eds) *Crime and Society: Readings in History and Theory*, Milton Keynes: Open University Press.

Hekman, S. (1990) *Gender and Knowledge: Elements of a Postmodern Feminism*, Cambridge: Polity Press.

Heller, T., Reynolds, J., Gomm, R., Muston, R. and Pattison, S. (eds) (1996) *Mental Health Matters: A Reader*, Basingstoke: Macmillan, in association with the Open University.

Henwood, M. (1990) *Community Care and Elderly People*, London: Family Policy Studies Centre.

Heraud, B.J. (1970) *Sociology and Social Work: Perspectives and Problems*, Oxford: Pergamon Press.

Herbert, M. (1997) 'Adolescence', in M. Davies (ed.) *The Blackwell Companion to Social Work*, Oxford: Blackwell.

Heron, C. (1998) *Working with Carers*, London: Jessica Kingsley.

Hester, S. and Eglin, P. (1992) *A Sociology of Crime*, London: Routledge.

Hill, M. (1987) *Sharing Child Care in Early Parenthood*, London: Routledge and Kegan Paul.

Hill, M. and Aldgate, J. (eds) (1996) *Child Welfare Services: Developments in Law, Policy, Practice and Research*, London: Jessica Kingsley.

Hill, M. and Tisdall, K. (1997) *Children and Society*, Harlow, Essex: Addison Wesley Longman Ltd.

Hill Collins, P. (1990) *Black Feminist Thought*, London: Harper Collins.

Hillery, G.A. (1955) 'Definitions of community: areas of agreement', *Rural Sociology* 20 Edition, (2): 111–23.

Hirschi, T. (1969) *Causes of Delinquency*, Berkeley: University of California Press.

Hochschild, A. (1990) *The Second Shift: Working Parents and the Revolution at Home*, New York: Viking Press.

Hockey, J. and James, A. (1993) *Growing Up and Growing Old: Ageing and Dependency in the Life Course*, London: Sage.

Holman, B. (1988) *Putting Families First: Prevention and Child Care*, Basingstoke: Macmillan.

Home Office (1984) *Probation Service in England and Wales: Statement of National Objectives and Priorities*, London: HMSO.

——(1992) *National Standards for the Supervision of Offenders in the Community*, London: HMSO.

——(1995) *National Standards for the Supervision of Offenders in the Community*, London: HMSO.

——(1999) *The Stephen Lawrence Inquiry: Report of an Inquiry by Sir William McPherson of Cluny*, London: HMSO.

Howe, D. (1987) *An Introduction to Social Work Theory*, Aldershot: Ashgate.

——(1991) 'The family and the therapist: Towards a sociology of social work method', in M. Davies (ed.) *The Sociology of Social Work*, London: Routledge.

——(1994) 'Modernity, postmodernity and social work', *British Journal of Social Work*, 24: 513–32.

Hudson, A. (1988) 'Boys will be boys: masculinism and the juvenile justice system', *Critical Social Policy* 21: 30–48.

——(1989) ' "Troublesome girls": Towards alternative definitions and policies', in M. Cain (ed.) *Growing up Good: Policing the Behaviour of Girls in Europe*, London: Sage.

Hudson, B. (1984) 'Femininity and adolescence', in A. McRobbie and M. Nava (eds) *Gender and Generation*, Basingstoke: Macmillan.

Huff, D. (1973) *How to Lie with Statistics*, Harmondsworth: Penguin.

Humphries, S. (1981) *Hooligan or Rebels?*, Oxford: Blackwell.

Irwin, S. (1995) 'Social reproduction and change in the transition from youth to adulthood', *Sociology* 29 (2): 293–316.

James, A. and Prout, A. (1990) *Constructing and Reconstructing Childhood: Contemporary Issues in the Sociological Study of Childhood*, London: Falmer Press.

Jamieson, L. and Toynbee, C. (1990) 'Shifting patterns of parental control', in H. Corr and L. Jamieson (eds) *The Politics of Everyday Life*, Basingstoke: Macmillan.

——(1992) *Country Bairns: Growing Up 1900–1930*, Edinburgh: Edinburgh University Press.

Jefferson, T. (1992) 'Wheelin' and stealin' ', *Achilles Heel* (13): 10–12.

Jenks, C. (1996) *Childhood*, London: Routledge.

Johnson, N. (1995) 'Domestic violence: An overview', in P. Kingston and B. Penhale (eds) *Family Violence and the Caring Professions*, Basingstoke: Macmillan.

Jones, C. (1997) 'British social work and the classless society: the failure of a profession', in H. Jones (ed.) *Towards a Classless Society?*, London: Routledge.

Jones, G. (1997) 'Youth homelessness and the 'underclass', in R. MacDonald (ed.) *Youth, the 'Underclass' and Social Exclusion*, London: Routledge.

Jones, G. and Wallace, C. (1992) *Youth, Family and Citizenship*, Buckingham: Open University Press.

Jones, H. (1997) *Towards a Classless Society?*, London: Routledge.

Jones, K., Brown, J. and Bradshaw, J. (1978) *Issues in Social Policy*, London: Routledge and Kegan Paul.

Jordan, B. (1996) *A Theory of Poverty and Social Exclusion*, Cambridge: Polity Press.

Kelly, L. (1988) *Surviving Sexual Violence*, Cambridge: Polity Press.

Kelly, L., Burton, S. and Regan, L. (1994) 'Researching women's lives or studying women's oppression? Reflections on what constitutes feminist research', in M. Maynard and J. Purvis (eds) *Researching Women's Lives from a Feminist Perspective*, London: Taylor and Francis.

Kelly, L., Wingfield, R., Burton, S. and Regan, L. (1995) *Splintered Lives: Sexual Exploitation of Children in the Context of Children's Rights and Child Protection*, London: Barnardo's.

Kemshall, H. (1995) 'Feminist criminology and probation practice: the implications for teaching DipSW probation courses', *Social Work Education* 14 (3): 79–93.

Kitzinger, J. (1990) 'Who are you kidding? Children and sociology in the UK', in L. Chisholm, P. Buchner, H. Kruger and P. Brown (eds) *Childhood, Youth and Social Change: A Comparative Perspective*, London: Falmer Press.

Klein, D.M. and White, J.M. (1996) *Family Theories: An Introduction*, London and California: Sage.

Knuttila, M. (1996) *Introducing Sociology: A Critical Perspective*, Ontario: Oxford University Press.

Kohlberg, L. (1981) *The Philosophy of Moral Development*, San Francisco: Harper Row.

Kumar, K. (1995) *From Post-Industrial to Post-Modern Society: New Theories of the Contemporary World*, Oxford: Basil Blackwell.

Langan, M. and Day, L. (eds) (1992) *Women, Oppression and Social Work: Issues in Anti-discriminatory Practice*, London: Routledge.

Lasch, C. (1977) *Haven in a Heartless World*, New York: Basic Books.

Laslett, T.P. (1972) 'Mean household size in England since the 16th century', in T.P. Laslett and R. Wall (eds) *Household and the Family in Past Time*, Cambridge: Cambridge University Press.

Leach, E. (1967) *A Runaway World*, London: BBC Publications.

Leat, D. and Gay, P. (1987) *Paying for Care*, Report 661, London: Policy Studies Institute.

Lee, M. and O'Brien, R. (1995) *The Game's Up*, London: The Children's Society.

Lees, S. (1986) *Losing Out: Sexuality and Adolescent Girls*, London: Hutchinson.

Lemert, E.M. (1951) *Social Pathology*, New York: McGraw-Hill.

——(1971) *Instead of Court*, Washington, DC: National Institute of Mental Health.

Leonard, P. (1966) *Sociology in Social Work*, London: Routledge and Kegan Paul.

——(1997) *Postmodern Welfare: Reconstructing an Emancipatory Project*, London: Sage.

Levitt, I. (1988) *Poverty and Welfare in Scotland 1890–1948*, Edinburgh: Edinburgh University Press.

Lewis, J. and Meredith, B. (1988) *Daughters Who Care Alone*, London: Routledge.

Lewis, O. (1949) *Life in a Mexican Village*, Illinois: Urbana, University of Illinois Press.

McCrone, D. (1992, 2002) *Understanding Scotland: The Sociology of a Stateless Nation*, London: Routledge.

MacDonald, R. (ed.) (1997) *Youth, the 'Underclass' and Social Exclusion*, London: Routledge.

Macfarlane, A. (1996) 'Aspects of intervention: consultation, care, help and support', in G. Hales (ed.) *Beyond Disability: Towards an Enabling Environment*, London: Sage, in association with the Open University.

McIntosh, M. (1979) 'The welfare state and the needs of the dependent family', in S. Burnam (ed.) *Fit Work for Women*, London: Croom Helm.

——(1996) 'Social anxieties about lone motherhood and ideologies of the family: Two sides of the same coin', in E. B. Silva (ed.) *Good Enough Mothering? Feminist Perspectives on Lone Motherhood*, London: Routledge.

Macionis, J.J. and Plummer, K. (1997) *Sociology: A Global Introduction*, New Jersey: Prentice Hall.

Mackie, M. (1987) *Constructing Men and Women: Gender Socialisation*, Canada: Holt, Rinehart and Winston.

McMillan, D.W. and Chavis, D.M. (1986) 'Sense of community: A definition and theory', *Journal of Community Psychology*, 14: 6–23.

McPherson, W. (1999) *Report into the Stephen Lawrence Enquiry*.

McRobbie, A. and Garber, J. (1976) 'Girls and subcultures', in S. Hall and T. Jefferson (eds) *Resistance through Rituals: Youth Subcultures in Post-War Britain*, London: Hutchinson and CCCS, University of Birmingham.

Maguire, M., Morgan, R. and Reiner, R. (eds) (1997) *The Oxford Handbook of Criminology*, Second edition, Oxford: Clarendon Press.

Mahood, L. (1995) *Policing Gender, Class and Family: Britain, 1850–1940*, London: UCL Press.

Marsh, I., Keating, M., Eyre, A., Campbell, R. and McKenzie, J. (1996) *Making Sense of Society: An Introduction to Sociology*, Harlow, Essex: Addison Wesley Longman.

Marsland, D. (1987) *Education and Youth*, London: Falmer Press.

Martin, J. and Roberts, C. (1984) *Women and Employment: A Lifetime Perspective*, London: HMSO.

Marx, K. and Engels, F. (1976) *Collected Works*, London: Lawrence and Wishart.

Matza, D. and Sykes, G. (1961) 'Juvenile delinquency and subterranean values', *American Sociological Review* 26: 712–19.

Mayall, B. (1994) *Children's Childhoods: Observed and Experienced*, London: Falmer Press.

——(1996) *Children, Health and the Social Order*, Buckingham: Open University Press.

Maynard, M. (1985) 'The response of social workers to domestic violence', in J. Pahl (ed.) *Private Violence and Public Policy*, London: Routledge and Kegan Paul.

——(1990) 'The re-shaping of sociology? Trends in the study of gender', *Sociology* 24 (2): 269–90.

230 Bibliography

Mead, G.H. (1934) *Mind, Self and Society*, Chicago: Chicago University Press.

Mead, M. (1928) *Coming of Age in Samoa*, London: Penguin.

Merton, R. (1957) *Social Theory and Social Structure*, New York: Free Press.

Meyerson, S. (1975) *Adolescence: The Crises of Adjustment*, London: George Allen and Unwin.

Mills, C.W. (1959) *The Sociological Imagination*, Oxford: Oxford University Press.

Mills, D. (1996) 'Community and nation in the past: perception and reality', in M. Drake (ed.) *Time, Family and Community: Perspectives on Family and Community History*, Oxford: Blackwell.

Moore, L. (1993) 'Educating for the woman's sphere', in E. Breitenbach and E. Gordon (eds) *Out of Bounds*, Edinburgh: Edinburgh University Press.

Morgan, D.H.J. (1975) *Social Theory and the Family*, London: Routledge and Kegan Paul.

Morgan, P. (1995) *Farewell to the Family*, London: Institute of Economic Affairs.

Morris, J. (1991) *Pride against Prejudice: Transforming Attitudes to Disability*, London: Women's Press.

——(1995) 'Creating a space for absent voices: disabled women's experience of receiving assistance with daily living activities', *Feminist Review* 51: 68–93.

——(1997) ' "Us" and "them"? Feminist research and community care', in J. Bornat, J. Johnson, C. Pereira, D. Pilgrim and F. Williams (eds) *Community Care: A Reader*, Second edition, Basingstoke: Macmillan and Open University.

——(1997) 'A response to Aldridge and Becker – "Disability rights and the denial of young carers: the danger of zero-sum arguments"', *Critical Social Policy* 17: 133–5.

Mouzelis, N. (1995) *Sociological Theory: What Went Wrong? Diagnosis and Remedies*, London: Routledge.

Mullender, A. (1996) *Rethinking Domestic Violence: The Social Work and Probation Response*, London: Routledge.

——(1997) 'Gender', in M. Davies (ed.) *The Blackwell Companion to Social Work*, Oxford: Blackwell.

Muncie, J. (1999) *Youth and Crime: A Critical Introduction*, London: Sage.

Muncie, J. and FitzGerald, M. (1981) 'Humanising the deviant: Affinity and affiliation theories', in M. FitzGerald, G. McLennan and J. Pawson (eds) *Crime and Society: Readings in History and Theory*, Milton Keynes: Open University Press.

Muncie, J., McLaughlin, E. and Langan, M. (1996) *Criminological Perspectives: A Reader*, London: Sage and Open University.

Muncie, J. and Sapsford, R. (1995) 'Issues in the study of "the family"', in J. Muncie, M. Wetherell, R. Dallos and A. Cochrane (eds) *Understanding the Family*, London: Open University and Sage.

Muncie, J. and Wetherell, M. (1995) 'Family policy and political discourse', in J. Muncie, M. Wetherell, R. Dallos and A. Cochrane (eds) *Understanding the Family*, London: Open University and Sage.

Muncie, J., Wetherall, M., Dallos, R. and Cochrane, A. (1995) *Understanding the Family*, London: Sage.

Murdock, G.P. (1965) *Social Structure*, Second edition, New York: Free Press.

Murray, C. (1990) *The Emerging British Underclass*, London: Institute of Economic Affairs, Health and Welfare Unit.

——(1993) 'The time has come to put a stigma back on illegitimacy', *Wall Street Journal*, 14 November.

Musgrave, P. (1972) *The Sociology of Education*, Second edition, London: Methuen.

Musgrove, F. (1968) *Youth and the Social Order*, London: Routledge and Kegan Paul.

Naffine, N. (1987) *Female Crime: The Construction of Women in Criminology*, London: Allen and Unwin.

Nava, M. (1983) 'From utopianism to scientific feminism', in L. Segal (ed.) *What Is To Be Done about the Family?*, Harmondsworth: Penguin.

——(1984) 'Youth service provision, social order and the question of girls', in A. McRobbie and M. Nava (eds) *Gender and Generation*, Basingstoke: Macmillan.

Nazroo, J. (1999) 'Uncovering gender differences in the use of marital violence: the effect of methodology', in G. Allan (ed) *The Sociology of the Family: A Reader*, Oxford: Blackwell.

Newburn, T. and Stanko, E.A. (1994) 'When men are victims: the failure of victimology', in T. Newburn and E.A. Stanko (eds) *Just Boys Doing Business: Men, Masculinities and Crime*, London: Routledge.

Newman, T. (1996) 'Rights, rites and responsibilities', in H. Roberts and D. Sachdev (eds) *Young People's Social Attitudes: Having their Say: the Views of 12–19 Year Olds*, London: Barnardo's.

Nissel, M. and Bonnerjea, L. (1982) *Family Care of the Handicapped Elderly: Who Pays?*, London: Policy Studies Institute.

Oakley, A. (1972) *Sex, Gender and Society*, London: Temple Smith.

——(1974) *The Sociology of Housework*, London: Martin Robertson.

Office for National Statistics (1996) *Social Focus on Ethnic Minorities*, London: HMSO.

Oldman, D. (1994) 'Adult–child relations as class realtions', in J. Qvortrup, M. Bardy, G. Sgritta and H. Wintersberger (eds) *Childhood Matters: Social Theory, Practice and Politics*, Aldershot: Avebury.

Oliver, M. (1990) *The Politics of Disablement*, Basingstoke: Macmillan.

Olsen, R. (1996) 'Young carers: challenging the facts and politics of research into children and caring', *Disability and Society* 11(1): 41–54.

Opie, I. (1993) *The People in the Playground*, Oxford: Oxford University Press.

Osgerby, B. (1998) *Youth in Britain since 1945*, Oxford: Blackwell.

Park, R.E. (1936) 'Human ecology', *American Journal of Sociology* 42 (1): 15.

Park, R.E., Burgess, E. and Mackenzie, R. (1923) *The City*, Chicago, IL: University of Chicago Press.

Parker, G. (1990) *With Due Care and Attention: A Review of Research on Informal Care*, Second edition, London: Family Policy Studies Centre.

Parker, G. and Lawton, D. (1994) *Different Types of Care, Different Types of Carer*, London: HMSO.

Parker, R. (1981) 'Tending and social policy', in E.M. Goldberg and S. Hatch (eds) *A New Look at the Personal Social Services*, Discussion Paper 4, London: Policy Studies Institute.

Parker, R., Ward, H., Jackson, S., Aldgate, J. and Wedge, P. (1991) *Assessing Outcomes in Child Care: Looking after Children*, London: HMSO.

Parsons, T. (1949) 'The social structure of the family', in R. N. Anshen (ed.) (1983) *The Family, Its Functions and Destiny*, New York: Harper.

——(1951, 1964) *The Social System*, New York: Free Press.

——(1955) 'The American family: its relation to personality and the social structure', in T. Parsons and R.F. Bales (eds) *Family Socialisation and Interaction Process*, New York: Free Press.

Parton, N. (1985) *The Politics of Child Abuse*, Basingstoke: Macmillan.

——(1991) *Governing the Family: Child Care, Child Protection and the State*, Basingstoke: Macmillan.

——(1994) 'Problematics of government, (post) modernity and social work', *British Journal of Social Work*, 24: 9–32.

——(ed.) (1996) *Social Theory, Social Change and Social Work*, London: Routledge.

Parton, N., Thorpe, D. and Wattam, C. (eds) (1997) *Child Protection: Risk and Moral Order*, Basingstoke: Macmillan.

Patel, N. (1990) *'Race' against Time: Social Services Provision to Black Elders*, London: Runnymede Trust.

Payne, C. (1994) 'The systems approach', in C. Hanvey and T. Philpot (eds) *Practising Social Work*, London: Routledge.

Payne, M. (1995) *Social Work and Community Care*, Basingstoke: Macmillan.

Pearson, G. (1983) *Hooligan: A History of Respectable Fears*, Basingstoke: Macmillan.

Pease, B. and Fook, J. (eds) (1999) *Transforming Social Work Practice*, London and Australia: Routledge and Allen and Unwin.

Perelberg, R.J. and Miller, A.C. (1990) *Gender and Power in Families*, London: Routledge.

Perring, C., Twigg, J. and Atkin, K. (1990) *Families Caring for People Diagnosed as Mentally Ill: the Literature Re-examined*, London: HMSO.

Phillips, A. (1993) *The Trouble with Boys*, London: Pandora.

Phillipson, C. and Biggs, S. (1995) 'Elder abuse: a critical overview', in P. Kingston and B. Penhale (eds) *Family Violence and the Caring Professions*, Basingstoke: Macmillan.

Pilcher, J. (1995) *Age and Generation in Modern Britain*, Oxford: Oxford University Press.

Pollock, L. (1987) *A Lasting Relationship: Parents and Children over Three Centuries*, London: Fourth Estate.

Pontin, D.J.T. (1988) 'The use of profile similarity indices and the Bem Sex Role Inventory in determining the sex role characterisation of a group of male and female nurses', *Journal of Advanced Nursing* 13: 768–74.

Postman, N. (1983) *The Disappearance of Childhood*, London: W.H. Allen.

Pringle, K. (1996) *Men, Masculinities and Social Welfare*, London: UCL Press.

——(1998) *Children and Social Welfare in Europe*, Buckingham: Open University Press.

Qureshi, H. and Walker, A. (1989) *The Caring Relationship*, Basingstoke: Macmillan.

Qvortrup, J. (1994) 'Childhood matters: An introduction', in J. Qvortrup, M. Bardy, G. Sgritta and H. Wintersberger (eds) *Childhood Matters: Social Theory, Practice and Politics*, Aldershot: Avebury.

——(1995) 'Childhood and modern society: a paradoxical relationship?', in J. Brannen and M. O'Brien (eds) *Childhood and Parenthood*, London: Institute of Education, University of London.

Ramazanoglu, C. (1989) *Feminism and the Contradictions of Oppression*, London: Routledge.

——(1993) *Up Against Foucault: Explorations of Some Tensions between Foucault and Feminism*, London: Routledge.

Rank, M.R. and Kain, E.L. (1995) *Diversity and Change in Families: Patterns, Prospects and Policies*, Englewood Cliffs, NJ: Prentice Hall.

Raynor, P. (1993) *Social Work, Justice and Control*, London: Whiting and Birch.

Redfield, R. (1947) 'The folk society', *American Journal of Sociology* 52 (3): 293–308.

Redhead, S. (1990) *The End-of-the-Century-Party: Youth and Pop toward 2000*, Manchester: Manchester University Press.

Rees, S. (1978) *Social Work Face to Face*, London: Edward Arnold.

Reiss, I.L. (1965) 'The universality of the family', *Journal of Marriage and the Family* 27 (November): 443–53.

Rex, J. and Moore, R. (1967) *Race, Community and Conflict: A Study of Sparkbrook*, Oxford: Oxford University Press.

Richmond, M. (1917) *Social Diagnosis*, New York: Russell Sage Foundation.

Ritzer, G. (1992) *Sociological Theory*, Third edition, New York: McGraw-Hill.

Roberts, E. (1996) 'Women and the domestic economy 1890–1970: the oral evidence', in M. Drake (ed.) *Time, Family and Community: Perspectives on Family and Community History*, Oxford: Blackwell.

Roberts, H. and Sachdev, D. (1996) *Young People's Social Attitudes: Having their Say: the Views of 12–19 Year Olds*, London: Barnardo's.

Roberts, K. (1995) *Youth and Employment in Modern Britain*, Oxford: Oxford University Press.

——(1997) 'Is there an emerging British "underclass"? The evidence from youth research', in R. MacDonald (ed.) *Youth, the 'Underclass' and Social Exclusion*, London: Routledge.

Robinson, L. (1995) *Psychology for Social Workers: Black Perspectives*, London: Routledge.

——(1997) 'Nigrescence', in M. Davies (ed.) *The Blackwell Companion to Social Work*, Oxford: Blackwell.

Rock, P. (1997) 'Sociological theories of crime', in M. Maguire, R. Morgan and R. Reiner (eds) *The Oxford Handbook of Criminology*, Second edition, Oxford: Clarendon Press.

Rodger, J.J. (1996) *Family Life and Social Control: A Sociological Perspective*, Basingstoke: Macmillan.

Rogers, A., Pilgrim, D. and Lacey, R. (1993) *Experiencing Psychiatry: Users' Views of Services*, Basingstoke: Macmillan, in association with MIND.

Rogers, W.S. (1989) 'Effective co-operation in child protection work', in S. Morgan and P. Righton (eds) *Child Care: Concerns and Conflicts*, London: Hodder and Stoughton.

Rose, N. (1993) 'Government, authority and expertise in advanced liberalism', *Economy and Society* 22 (3): 283–99.

Rowbotham, S. (1973) *Women's Consciousness, Man's World*, Harmondsworth: Penguin.

Rudd, P. and Evans, K. (1998) 'Structure and agency in youth transitions: Student experiences of vocational higher education', *Journal of Youth Studies* 1 (1): 39–62.

Russell, G. (1983) *The Changing Role of Fathers*, Milton Keynes: Open University Press.

Rutter, M., Graham, P., Chadwick, O.F.D. and Yule, W. (1976) 'Adolescent turmoil: fact of fiction?', *Journal of Child Psychology and Psychiatry* 17: 35–56.

Saporiti, A. (1994) 'A methodology for making children count', in J. Qvortrup, M. Bardy, G. Sgritta and H. Wintersberger (eds) *Childhood Matters: Social Theory, Practice and Politics*, Aldershot: Avebury.

Saussure, F. de (1974) *Course in General Linguistics*, London: Fontana.

Schon, D.A. (1983) *The Reflective Practitioner: How Professionals Think in Action*, London: Temple Smith.

Schutz, A. (1976) *The Phenomenology of the Social World*, London: Heinemann.

Scottish Office Social Work Services Group (1991) *National Objectives and Standards for Social Work Services in the Criminal Justice System*, Edinburgh: The Scottish Office Social Work Services Group.

——(1996) *National Guidelines on Diversion to Social Work and Other Service Agencies as an Alternative to Prosecution*, Edinburgh: The Scottish Office Social Work Services Group.

Scourfield, J.B. (1998) 'Probation officers working with men', *British Journal of Social Work* 28 (4): 581–600.

Scraton, P. (ed.) (1997) *'Childhood' in 'Crisis'?*, London: UCL Press.

Scraton, P. and Chadwick, K. (1991) 'The theoretical and political priorities of critical criminology', in K. Stenson and D. Cowell (eds) *The Politics of Crime Control*, London: Sage.

Segal, L. (1983) *What Is To Be Done about the Family?*, Harmondsworth: Penguin.

——(1990) *Slow Motion: Changing Masculinities*, London: Virago.

Sennett, R. (1977) *The Fall of Public Man*, Cambridge: Cambridge University Press.

——(1980) 'Destructive gemeinschaft', reprinted in R. Bocock, P. Hamilton, K. Thompson and A. Waton (eds) *An Introduction to Sociology*, London: Fontana.

Sharpe, S. (1976) *Just Like a Girl*, Harmondsworth: Penguin.

Sheldon, B. (1986) 'Social work effectiveness experiments: Review and implications', *British Journal of Social Work* 17: 635–44.

Shoemaker, D.J. (1990) *Theories of Delinquency: An Examination of Explanations of Delinquent Behaviour*, New York: Oxford University Press.

Sibeon, R. (1991) *Towards a New Sociology of Social Work*, Aldershot: Avebury.

Simmel, G. (1971) 'The metropolis and mental life (1903)', in K. Thompson and J. Tunstall (eds) *Sociological Perspectives*, Penguin: Harmondsworth.

Smart, C. (1976) *Women, Crime and Criminology: A Feminist Critique*, London: Routledge and Kegan Paul.

——(1990) 'Feminist approaches to criminology or postmodern woman meets atavistic man', in L. Gelsthorpe and A. Morris (eds) *Feminist Perspectives in Criminology*, Buckingham: Open University Press.

Smart, C. and Smart, B. (1978) *Women, Sexuality and Social Control*, London: Routledge and Kegan Paul.

Smith, C. and White, S. (1997) 'Parton, Howe and postmodernity: A critical comment on mistaken identity', *British Journal of Social Work*, 27: 275–95.

Smith, D. (1988) *The Everyday World as Problematic*, Milton Keynes: Open University Press.

Smith, D.J. (1995) *Criminology for Social Work*, Basingstoke: Macmillan.

——(1997) 'Ethnic origins, crime and criminal justice', in M. Maguire, R. Morgan and R. Reiner (eds) *The Oxford Handbook of Criminology*, Second edition, Oxford: Clarendon Press.

Smith, D.M. (1987) 'Peers, subcultures and schools', in D. Marsland (ed.) *Education and Youth*, London: Falmer Press.

Smith, M. (1965) *Professional Education for Social Work in Britain*, London: Allen and Unwin.

Social Work Services Inspectorate (1995) *Social Work Services in the Criminal Justice System: Achieving National Standards*, Edinburgh: The Scottish Office.

Springhall, J. (1986) *Coming of Age: Adolescence in Britain 1860–1960*, Dublin: Gill and Macmillan.

Stanley, L. (ed.) (1990) *Feminist Praxis: Research, Theory and Epistemology in Feminist Sociology*, London: Routledge.

Stets, J. (1988) *Domestic Violence and Control*, New York: Springer-Verlag.

Stewart, F. (1992) 'The adolescent as consumer', in J.C. Coleman and C. Warren-Adamson (eds) *Youth Policy in the 1990s: The Way Forward*, London: Routledge.

Straus, M.A. and Gelles, R.J. (1986) 'Societal change and change in family violence from 1975 to 1985 as revealed by two national surveys', *Journal of Marriage and the Family*, 48.

Sullivan, M. (1987) *Sociology and Social Welfare*, London: Unwin Hyman.

Sutherland, E.H. (1939) *Principles of Criminology*, Third edition, Philadelphia: Lippincott.

Sutherland, E.H. and Cressey, D.R. (1978) *Criminology*, Tenth edition, New York: Columbia University Press.

Swingewood, A. (1984) *A Short History of Sociological Thought*, London: Macmillan.

Syal, M. (1996) *Anita and Me*, London: Flamingo.

Symonds, A. (1998) 'Social construction and the concept of "community"', in A. Symonds and A. Kelly (eds) *The Social Construction of Community Care*, Basingstoke: Macmillan.

Tannenbaum, F. (1938) *Crime and Community*, New York: Columbia University.

Taylor, I., Walton, P. and Young, J. (1975) *Critical Criminology*, London: Routledge and Kegan Paul.

Tester, S. (1996) 'Women and community care', in C. Hallett (ed.) *Women and Social Policy: An Introduction*, London: Harvester Wheatsheaf.

Thane, P. (1981) 'Childhood in history', in M. King (ed.) *Childhood, Welfare and Justice: A Critical Examination of Children in the Legal and Childcare Systems*, London: Batsford.

Thomas, C. (1993) 'De-constructing concepts of care', *Sociology* 27 (4): 649–69.

Thompson, P. (1981) 'Life histories and the analysis of social change', in D. Bertaux (ed.) *Biography and Society*, Beverly Hills: Sage.

Thompson, N. (1997) *Anti-Discriminatory Practice,* Second edition, Macmillan: Basingstoke.

Thorogood, N. (1987) 'Race, class and gender. The politics of housework', in Brannen, J. and Wilson, G. (eds) *Give and Take in Families*, London: Allen and Unwin.

Tisdall, K. (1996) 'From the Social Work (Scotland) Act 1968 to the Children (Scotland) Act 1995: pressures for change', in M. Hill and J. Aldgate (eds) *Child Welfare Services. Developments in Law, Policy, Practice and Research*, London: Jessica Kingsley.

Tizard, B. and Phoenix, A. (1993) *Black, White or Mixed Race? Race and Racism in the Lives of Young People of Mixed Parentage*, London: Routledge.

Tolson, A. (1977) *The Limits of Masculinity*, London: Tavistock.

Tonnies, F. (1955) *Community and Association (1887)*, London: Routledge and Kegan Paul.

Townsend, P. (1962) *The Last Refuge*, London: Routledge and Kegan Paul.

Triseliotis, J. (1980) *New Developments in Adoption and Foster Care*, London: Routledge and Kegan Paul.

Tuson, G. (1996) 'Writing postmodern social work', in P. Ford and P. Hayes (eds) *Educating for Social Work: Arguments for Optimism*, Aldershot: Avebury.

Ulas, M. and Connor, A. (eds) (1999) *Mental Health and Social Work*, London: Jessica Kingsley.

Ungerson, C. (1983) 'Why do women care?', in J. Finch and D. Groves (eds) *A Labour of Love: Women, Work and Caring*, London: Routledge and Kegan Paul.

Ussher, J. (ed.) (1997) *Body Talk*, London: Routledge.

Van Den Haag, E. (1975) *Punishing Criminals*, New York: Simon and Schuster.

Vasey, S. (1996) 'The experience of care', in G. Hales (ed.) *Beyond Disability: Towards an Enabling Environment*, London: Sage, in association with the Open University.

Walby, S. (1990) *Theorising Patriarchy*, Oxford: Blackwell.

Walklate, S. (1989) *Victimology*, London: Unwin Hyman.

Wall, R. (1992) 'Relationships between generations in British families past and present', in C. Marsh and S. Arber (eds) *Families and Households: Divisions and Change*, Basingstoke: Macmillan.

Wallace, C. (1987) 'Between the family and the state: young people in transition', in M. White (ed.) *The Social World of the Young Unemployed*, London: Policy Studies Institute.

Waterhouse, L., Dobash, R. and Carnie, J. (1994) *Child Sexual Abusers*, Edinburgh: The Scottish Office.

Waterhouse, L. and McGhee, J. (1996) 'Families', social workers' and police perspectives on child abuse investigations', in M. Hill and J. Aldgate (eds) *Child Welfare Services: Developments in Law, Policy, Practice and Research*, London: Jessica Kingsley.

Waterhouse, L. (1997) 'Child abuse', in M. Davies (ed.) *The Blackwell Companion to Social Work*, Oxford: Blackwell.

Weber, M. (1974) *The Protestant Ethic and the Spirit of Capitalism*, London: Unwin.

Weedon, C. (1987) *Feminist Practice and Post-structuralist Theory*, Oxford: Blackwell.

Weeks, J. (1986) *Sexuality*, London: Tavistock.

Weeks, J., Heaphy, B. and Donovan, C. (1999) 'Partners by choice: equality, power and commitment in non-heterosexual relationships', in G. Allan (ed.) *The Sociology of the Family: A Reader*, Oxford: Blackwell.

White, M. (1988) *And Grandmother's Bed Went Too: Poor But Happy in Somers Town*, London: St Pancras Housing Association, Camden.

Whyte, B. (1998) 'Rediscovering juvenile delinquency', in A. Lockyer and F.H. Stone (eds) *Juvenile Justice in Scotland: Twenty-Five Years of the Welfare Approach*, Edinburgh: T. and T. Clark.

Wilczynski, A. (1995) 'Child-killing by parents: social, legal and gender issues', in R.E. Dobash, R.P. Dobash and L. Noaks (eds) *Gender and Crime*, Cardiff: University of Wales Press.

Williams, F. (1997) 'Women and community', in J. Bornat, J. Johnson, C. Pereira, D. Pilgrim and F. Williams (eds) *Community Care: A Reader*, Second edition, Basingstoke: Macmillan and Open University.

Willis, P. (1977) *Learning to Labour*, Farnborough: Saxon House.

——(1990) *Common Culture: Symbolic Work at Play in the Everyday Cultures of the Young*, Milton Keynes: Open University Press.

Wilson, E. (1982) 'Women, the "community" and the "family" ', in A. Walker (ed.) *Community Care: The Family, the State and Social Policy*, Oxford: Basil Blackwell/Martin Robertson.

——(1977) *Women and the Welfare State*, London: Tavistock.

Wilson, J. (1975) *Thinking about Crime*, New York: Basic Books.

Wilson, M. (1996) 'Working with the CHANGE men's programme', in K. Cavanagh and V.E. Cree (eds) *Working with Men: Feminism and Social Work*, London: Routledge.

Wirth, L. (1938) 'Urbanism as a way of life', *American Journal of Sociology* 44 (1): 1–24.

Wright, F.D. (1986) *Left to Care Alone*, Aldershot: Gower.

Wrong, D.H. (1961) 'The over-socialised conception of man in modern sociology', *American Sociological Review* 26 (April): 183–93.

Yelloly, M.A. (1980) *Social Work Theory and Psychoanalysis*, New York: Van Nostrand Reinhold.

Young, J. (1981) 'Thinking seriously about crime: some models of criminology', in M. Fitzgerald, G. McLennan and J. Pawson (eds) *Crime and Society: Readings in History and Theory*, London: Routledge and Kegan Paul.

——(1986) 'The failure of criminology: the need for a radical realism', in R. Matthews and J. Young (eds) *Confronting Crime*, London: Sage.

Young, M. and Willmott, P. (1957) *Family and Kinship in East London*, London: Routledge and Kegan Paul.

——(1975) *The Symmetrical Family*, Harmondsworth: Penguin.

Zaretsky E. (1976) *Capitalism, the Family and Personal Life*, London: Pluto Press.

Name Index

Subject Index

U.W.E.L LEARNING RESOURCES